In Search of Sexual Health

In Search of Sexual Health

DIAGNOSING AND TREATING SYPHILIS
IN HOT SPRINGS, ARKANSAS
1890–1940

Elliott Bowen

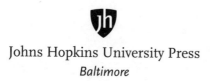

Johns Hopkins University Press
Baltimore

© 2020 Johns Hopkins University Press
All rights reserved. Published 2020
Printed in the United States of America on acid-free paper

2 4 6 8 9 7 5 3 1

Johns Hopkins University Press
2715 North Charles Street
Baltimore, Maryland 21218-4363
www.press.jhu.edu

Library of Congress Cataloging-in-Publication Data

Names: Bowen, Elliott G., 1983– author.
Title: In search of sexual health : Diagnosing and treating syphilis
   in Hot Springs, Arkansas, 1890–1940 / Elliot Bowen.
Description: Baltimore : Johns Hopkins University Press, [2020] |
   Includes bibliographical references and index.
Identifiers: LCCN 2019047601 | ISBN 9781421438566 (hardcover) |
   ISBN 9781421438573 (ebook)
Subjects: LCSH: Army and Navy General Hospital (Hot Springs, Ark.) |
   United States. Public Health Service. Division of Venereal Diseases. |
   Syphilis—Treatment—Arkansas—Hot Springs—History. |
   Hospitals—Arkansas—Hot Springs—History. |
   Soldiers—Health and hygiene—United States—History.
Classification: LCC RC201.5.A8 B89 2020 | DDC 616.95/1300976741—dc23
LC record available at https://lccn.loc.gov/2019047601

A catalog record for this book is available from the British Library.

*Special discounts are available for bulk purchases of this book. For more
information, please contact Special Sales at specialsales@press.jhu.edu.*

Johns Hopkins University Press uses environmentally friendly book materials,
including recycled text paper that is composed of at least 30 percent
post-consumer waste, whenever possible.

For my sister Emi, whose time came too soon

CONTENTS

For much of human history, syphilis, gonorrhea, and other sexually transmitted diseases have been regarded as taboo subjects—as things that, if discussed at all, are discussed only among close friends or intimate acquaintances. Thankfully, that has not been the case in the ten years I have spent researching and writing this book. Over the last decade, my thoughts about Hot Springs, Arkansas, and its experience with syphilis have benefited immensely from untold numbers of conversations with mentors, colleagues, archivists, friends, relatives, and fellow researchers. In settings both public and private, the ideas these individuals have shared with me have been of invaluable assistance—as has the support they've provided through what at times has been a very difficult, tumultuous journey from PhD dissertation to published monograph. In what follows, I would like to acknowledge some of the many individuals who have helped this project along at various stages of its development. Without their help, I simply would not be where I am today.

The research for this book began during my graduate school days at Binghamton University, New York. My first thanks thus go to my advisor, Jerry Kutcher, who not only guided me through this entire dissertation process but also, along the way, taught me how to be a historian of medicine. In addition to the stellar guidance I received as Jerry's student, I was also fortunate enough to have Leigh Ann Wheeler, Stephen Ortiz, and Fa-ti Fan on my PhD committee, and I would like to thank each of them for helping steer and shepherd my dissertation toward its completion. Working together, these extraordinarily skilled, wonderfully patient, and altogether selfless individuals graciously critiqued preliminary versions of my chapters, came to see me deliver conference papers and mock job talks, and advanced my thinking on Hot Springs' historical significance—even when the subject of my work veered away from their own areas of expertise. From the bottom of my heart, I thank each of you.

During my time at Binghamton, I also received the gracious support of both the Institute for Advanced Studies in the Humanities and the university's history department, whose combined financial largesse funded the archival trips required to complete the research for this book. While in Arkansas, I received extensive assistance from a number of incredibly friendly and resourceful archivists, each of whom (to my thankful surprise) had no qualms whatsoever when it came to discussing the ins and outs of syphilis's role in their state's history. Here I would first like to thank Liz Robbins of the Garland County Historical Society, who brought the papers of Archie A. Cowles to my attention. Tommy Hill of the National Park Service archives also made an immeasurable contribution to my research, as without his efforts I would have never located the correspondence of Michael J. Murphy. Finally, I would like to thank Amanda Saar at the University of Arkansas for Medical Sciences, who provided me access to the papers of Oliver C. Wenger and spent many an afternoon with me discussing interesting articles on syphilis from the *Journal of the Arkansas Medical Society*.

After graduating with my PhD in 2016, I was fortunate enough to find an academic job in the history of medicine at Nazarbayev University in Nur-Sultan (formerly Astana), Kazakhstan. In my three years here, this book has moved from dissertation to completed manuscript, and that transition has happened largely because of the generous support I've received from this institution. In addition to funding additional research trips and granting me ample time to revise this book's various chapters, employment at Nazarbayev University has allowed me to publish sections of my research as independent journal articles and to present parts of my work at on-campus gatherings and conferences all across the world. Beyond this, living and working in Central Asia brought me the love of my life, the person whose support, encouragement, and criticism helped me get this book across the finish line. To my partner, Erika Alpert, my dearest love: I owe you a debt that cannot be repaid.

Finally, I would like to thank my parents. Ever since I began my graduate studies at New Mexico State University in 2007, my mom and dad have supported my attempts to become a professional historian in myriad ways. Given that this was not my original career path, I want to thank both of you for sticking with me, for always being there for me, and for putting up with all the endless discussions about Hot Springs and its struggles with syphilis.

In Search of Sexual Health

Introduction

On March 14, 1897, a Baltimore man named G. W. Banks composed a lengthy letter to a woman named Genie. Opening his communiqué with news of a snowstorm that had recently blanketed the city, Banks then turned to more personal matters, detailing in quick succession his continued battles with rheumatism, visits from a student, and the great joy a canine companion named King brought him whenever his spirits sagged. Banks concluded with a bit of gossip he had learned from a West Virginia newspaper: two of his acquaintances, identified as Ross Hodges and Shepherd, had recently "gone to Hot Springs, Arkansas." The cause of their departure was no secret, Banks confided, though he commented that he wouldn't like it if his "town paper publish[ed] it if *I* had a Venereal Disease." Perhaps sensing that his reader required further clarification, Banks then placed the pair's dramatic disappearance in a broader context, explaining simply that "all syphalitics [*sic*] go to Hot Springs."[1]

Whether Hodges and Shepherd ever reached their destination is unknown. Had they done so, they would have been only two of some thirty thousand individuals to descend on Hot Springs in 1897, 70 percent of whom reportedly suffered from syphilis.[2] According to local physicians, Hot Springs was a city "where thousands come annually to be treated for syphilis," many from "hundreds of miles away."[3] Testifying to its popularity among sufferers of this venereal disease, one medical authority reported in the final decade of the nineteenth century on how "syphilitic subjects by the thousands flock to the place from all parts of the United States."[4] It was for these reasons that late nineteenth-century medical men began referring to Hot Springs as "a mecca for syphilitics in America."[5]

The city retained this status well into the new century. "We see every day, here in Hot Springs," one local physician noted in a 1913 treatise, "from ten to a hundred persons" suffering from the "terrible disease" that was syphilis.[6] Over the course of the next two decades, some sixty thousand syphilitic men and women traveled to this southern city for treatment, a phenomenon that prompted one resident observer to note that "to the average layman, Hot Springs, Arkansas, means VD, and VD means Hot Springs."[7] Only with the expanding availability of penicillin in the 1940s did this central Arkansas locale's status as a therapeutic refuge for syphilitics come to an end.

For more than a half century, much of the United States' struggle with sexually transmitted illness ran through Hot Springs. In addition to the thousands of health seekers who traveled there, the city was home to dozens of medical offices run by privately practicing venereal specialists, a military hospital whose surgeons treated the nation's syphilis-stricken soldiers and sailors, and a free VD clinic operated by the United States Public Health Service (PHS). Within these varied institutions, attempts to understand and overcome this debilitating disease took on an intensely local character. Despite considerable shifts in clinical practice during the nineteenth and twentieth centuries, Hot Springs' response to syphilis drew more on the interactions of visiting health seekers, resort doctors, and the city's permanent residents than it did on the writings of national medical authorities, the policies of the federal government, or the beliefs of prominent cultural figures. In an era in which coastal elites exercised increasing authority over all aspects of medical care, Hot Springs—a remote, fairly obscure town in the Ozark hinterlands—played a key role in determining treatment norms, attitudes, and parameters around syphilis. A local node with a significant national impact, Hot Springs offers a new perspective on a critical era in American medicine and public health.

In Search of Sexual Health

The importance of Hot Springs in treating syphilis coincided with an age of incipient health seeking. Though the term "medical tourism" is of recent coinage, the phenomenon it purports to describe is not a new one.[8] Ancient Greek healers such as Hippocrates (470–377 BCE) and Asclepiades (c. 124 BCE) introduced the idea of environmentally based cures and, in subsequent centuries, the fields of climatotherapy (treatment via change of climate) and balneotherapy (treatment via bathing) gradually blossomed.[9] During the colonial period of American history, settlers espoused a belief in "land health," maintaining that the boundaries between human bodies and the natural world were incredibly porous. At that time, prospective settlers commonly remarked on an area's salubrious or insalubrious status, crafting a geography of health that so tightly bound up disease and environment that both doctors and laypeople spoke of such maladies as "swamp fever" and "Arkansas chills."[10]

During the nineteenth century, this place-based understanding of health became increasingly medicalized, as doctor-scientists used instruments such as the thermometer, barometer, and hygrometer to measure seasonal patterns in temperature, humidity, cloudiness, and a variety of other climatic phenomena in locations all across the country.[11] From this budding interest in medical geography came studies like Henry Bowditch's *Consumption in America* (1869), which employed statistical methods to correlate the incidence of tuberculosis with climatological conditions in various regions.[12] On the basis of these investigations, health seeking became a recognized part of professional medicine, and with the completion of the transcontinental railroad in 1869, a "health rush" ensued.[13] Railroad promoters and local boosters trumpeted the health-giving qualities of the Rocky Mountains and the Great American Desert, inspiring consumptive "lungers" to seek out the warm, sunny climes of growing cities such as Denver, Tucson, and Santa Fe. In the decades following the Civil War, Americans "chasing the cure" also took to the mountainous forests of the Adirondacks, Vermont's White Mountains, and Michigan's Battle Creek Sanitarium, seeking treatment for all manner of diseases and in the process helping give rise to a curative industry organized around the health resort.[14] By the beginning of the twentieth century, the United States was awash in health resorts—many of which were located along rivers, watering holes, and other hydropathic hideaways.[15]

Uneasiness with the conditions of urban, industrial life provided a further stimulus to health seeking. Convinced that cities were inherently disease-ridden, pestilence-spreading places, Americans came to see *all* nonurban environments as healthful.[16] Those suffering from what Charles Rosenberg has termed "the pathologies of progress" increasingly pinned their hopes for restored health and happiness to the more natural environment of the countryside.[17]

In response, health resorts crafted a "diseases of civilization" narrative, deliberately targeting modernity's discontents—whether they were "brain-fagged" neurasthenics broken down from the stresses and demands of the city's maddening pace, swollen-eyed hay feverites who linked the city's pollen-free environment to their seasonal contractions of "autumnal catarrh," or lung-damaged consumptives who saw in the urban landscape the cause of the era's "great white plague."[18]

One of the most frequented of the era's health resorts was Saratoga Springs, a New York town whose waters were said to "run with an elixir of life" that offered rejuvenation to those suffering from diseases and disturbances "fostered by the pace of our modern, high-pressure civilization."[19] Also located in New York, the outdoor consumption clinic created by Edward L. Trudeau at Saranac

Lake similarly played into this "pathologies of progress" narrative, as its supporters noted how easily the "complexities of civilization" caused tubercular patients to forget that their health depended on the "simple great beneficial things of life," like "fresh air."[20] Coming into existence at a time when "modern civilization" had begun to work against the "natural development of mankind," Michigan's Battle Creek Sanitarium aimed to "teach people how to achieve natural modes of living under the changing conditions of modern life."[21] The common themes at Hot Springs and at other resorts were that "many of the conditions of modern life are distinctly unfavorable to health" and that specialized care of "all the serious ailments of modern life" could be found there.[22] The "camp cure" enjoyed great favor in the treatment of civilization's ills; medical authorities conceded that among those "great groups of diseases" that had their origins in "modern life," there was often no remedy superior to it.[23]

Though to date it has largely escaped scholarly attention, VD was one of the "pathologies of progress" that made medical tourism so popular in turn-of-the-century America. Contemporary physicians regularly encountered syphilitic patients convinced that their infections would remain uncured unless they went "to a thermomineral bathing place."[24] Citing hydrotherapy's "strong hold on the popular mind," venereal specialists heatedly debated its merits, with most upbraiding the laity for its belief in the "fallacious notion" that places like Hot Springs were a "cure all" for syphilis.[25] Yet despite their contention that the value of thermal and mineral springs were "very greatly overestimated," medical observers nevertheless conceded that in certain cases, such treatment greatly aided recovery.[26] As one prominent syphilographer explained, these waters possessed diuretic and diaphoretic properties that promoted the elimination of syphilitic poisons and those toxic chemicals (namely mercury and the iodides of potassium) necessary to its cure.[27] Because they had the ability to increase their ambulatory powers, doctors also regularly advised that patients afflicted with rheumatism, neuralgia, and paralysis caused by syphilis arrange a trip to the baths.[28]

Fueled by the popular belief that mineral and thermal springs offered a powerful means of antisyphilitic therapy, a number of health resorts dedicated to the treatment of this disease emerged in the late nineteenth century. Among the most popular was Hot Springs, South Dakota. Located in the Black Hills at a site thirty-four-hundred feet above sea level, this resort's spas, sanitariums, and hotels offered treatment in "syphilis and functional diseases of the liver and stomach."[29] Another popular option was French Lick Springs, Indiana, where doctors employed a local substance known as Pluto Water to treat syphilis and other "abnormal" conditions.[30]

While the aforementioned sites offered health seekers waters with an average temperature above 90 degrees Fahrenheit, a third resort used cold water therapies. This was Mt. Clemens, Michigan, where resident doctors boasted that syphilis "may be cured *by nature*, the patient taking no medicine."[31] Well into the early twentieth century, practitioners in Mt. Clemens observed that upward of 50 percent of the cases seen there were "of syphilitic origin," and nonresident healers noted instances of patients being given an "anti-syphilitic serum" in addition to hydrotherapeutic remedies.[32]

The Rocky Mountains also boasted sites of venereal therapy. The greatest fame in this region accrued to Glenwood Springs, Colorado, whose sulfur baths were said to have been used by pre-Columbian Native Americans "suffering from wounds of rheumatism or syphilis."[33] Taking the waters there, doctors averred, stimulated the sweat glands, enabling the patient to "throw off the poison" of syphilis through an increase in the elimination of mercury and potassium iodide. Such a method allowed patients to withstand "a much larger dose" of these chemicals.[34]

California, one of the country's most popular destinations for health seekers, was not lacking in antisyphilitic watering holes. In the Coahuila Valley, some fifty miles outside of San Diego, lay the Aguas Calientes, a "pleasant little resort" that possessed "infallible remedies in syphilis."[35] Another option was Gilroy Hot Springs; located in the Santa Clara Mountains, its alkalo-sulfurous waters were "used with considerable benefit in syphilis."[36] Lastly, a resort at Arrowhead Springs offered a "certain cure for syphilis" and was rumored to have been used "extensively" for that purpose by Native Americans "in former years."[37]

As these examples demonstrate, sexually transmitted diseases provided a significant stimulus to health travel in turn-of-the-century America. Knowing that "many syphilitics" would "demand hydrotherapy," some doctors took it upon themselves to study and classify the various health resorts available to those suffering from this disease and to publish information designed to aid colleagues in the selection of the proper destination for different types of syphilitic patients.[38] This was a matter of "decided import," as although some resorts offered the "proper advice and treatment," others were evidently rife with "fraud, quackery, and incompetency."[39]

Among the various resorts catering to individuals with syphilis, there was none that enjoyed a greater vogue than Hot Springs, Arkansas, which attracted more health seekers than all of its competitors combined.[40] Holding "the most prominent rank" among the various mineral and thermal springs of the country, it was an incredibly popular site for those hoping to get syphilis "boiled out" via hydrotherapy.[41] As one venereal specialist described it, "Patients with syphilis were very apt to get the idea that the only sure cure for their disease was at these springs, and were induced to return year after year."[42] Many insisted that syphilis could not be cured "save by a trip" there.[43]

Within Hot Springs, the "old, broken down" case of syphilis was especially on display. According to one turn-of-the-century visitor, the city's Central Avenue was a place where one met "all kinds of cripples and diseased human beings," venereally afflicted men who constantly trekked from boarding room to hotel to bathhouse and back again. "Here comes a man," he relayed,

> with the heels of his shoes shuffling the sidewalk, and the foot finally striking down in a manner that would suggest that he would not care if he kicked the front part of his foot from the tarsus attachments; he is a case of locomotor ataxia. There goes a man with one foot scraping the sidewalk, and a side motion of the body, with the arm and hand of the corresponding side making a full-stride. This is a case of hemiplegia, caused by syphilis. Here is a man with crutches, and he meanders slowly, and walks as though he were stepping on eggs; his joints are enlarged, and he is here working out a case of gonorrheal rheumatism. . . . [Here comes] the patient pushing his feet along, and with a cane in either hand, walking like a patient with a Potter's spine, is recovering from a lesion of the spinal cord, of syphilitic origin.

In addition to the movements of these syphilitic sufferers, one met in Hot Springs the daily journeys of the undertaker, who "with a pine box . . . returns a victim to his final resting place. Syphilis has again secured another victory."[44]

Why did so many Americans go "chasing the cure" for this disease? In particular, who were the individuals who came to Hot Springs in search of sexual health? Why did they go there, and what were their experiences like? More generally, how did the city's response to syphilis change over time, and how did Hot Springs both contribute to and reflect broader patterns of venereological care?

Medical matters such as these have not received adequate attention from historians of health tourism. Much of the scholarship on this topic revolves around three main themes: the growth of health tourism as a commercial industry, the patterns of settlement and community development this fostered, and the role resorts played as incubators of social relations and class hierarchies. A considerable, growing body of research has detailed the process by which individuals and institutions promoted medical travel (through advertising in newspapers and magazines, for example), how the expansion of railway networks (particularly the completion of the transcontinental railroad in 1869) facilitated this, how the increasing presence of tourists-cum-residents transformed upstart resort towns near mountainsides, natural springs, and other salubrious locations into full-fledged urban communities, and how a distinct "leisure class" emerged through the interactions of the social elites who often visited these luxurious establishments.[45] In connection with this last theme, historians have also illuminated the various strategies of exclusion state and municipal authorities made use of in order to prevent poor, socially disadvantaged health seekers from partaking of the naturopathic blessings of particular resort communities.[46] In addition to this, historians such as Gregg Mitman have shown how a combination of industrial development (mining and smelting, for example) and laboratory-derived medical technologies (especially antihistamines and corticosteroids) ultimately undermined the phenomenon affectionately referred to as "chasing the cure."[47]

Yet it remains somewhat unclear what this cure consisted of. Though in some cases, the basic elements of the curative regimens enacted at different resorts have been sketched out, by and large, neither the behaviors of health seekers nor their interactions with medical personnel have received much attention from historians. While promotional materials often stressed the benefits of outdoor living, dietary changes, rest, bathing and the cessation of such urban vices as tobacco and alcohol consumption, the question of what visiting patients actually did in order to recover from illness has not been sufficiently addressed. That is to say, many existing studies privilege the tourist side of "medical tourism" over the phenomenon's medical aspects. As a result, although investigations into this have yielded important insights regarding the emergence of "modern marketing techniques," much remains to be learned about how health resorts also contributed to the development of modern *therapeutic* techniques.[48]

The benefits of this line of inquiry can be seen from the work of Meghan Crnic and Cynthia Connolly.[49] In their analysis of late nineteenth- and early twentieth-century maritime children's hospitals, Crnic and Connolly elaborate on the various components of the "fresh air regimen" these pediatric facilities developed while caring for American youth who were sent to the Atlantic coast for treatment of tuberculosis. Most of the children admitted to these institutions were the sons and daughters of immigrants, and on account of the nativist sympathies of hospital staff, the program of clinical care administered sought not only to alleviate the symptoms of tuberculosis but also to inculcate "American" values (through Bible readings, prayer, and the consumption of middle-class dietary staples such as beef stew and mashed potatoes). The legacy of these seaside hospitals, Crnic and Connolly argue, can be seen in more recent initiatives like the Fresh Air Fund and the Hole in the Wall Camp Gang (a summer camp for children with cancer). As this research shows, exploring the therapeutic dimensions of medical tourism reveals much about the ideological assumptions that underwrote health-seeking behavior and about health care's sociocultural dimensions. It also brings to light the connections between programs of clinical management implemented at health resorts and more general contemporary medical developments.

In Search of Sexual Health engages with similar questions. Examining the history of Hot Springs from the perspective of medical practice, it exploits a unique source base that includes patient narratives, the private correspondence of individual health seekers, clinical case files, and the published and unpublished writings of Hot Springs' health care providers. Taken together, these materials uncover the constellation of social, cultural, economic, and political factors that shaped and reshaped patterns of clinical care within this singular site between the late nineteenth and early twentieth centuries. They also shed light on the development and evolution of antisyphilitic diagnostic and curative practices more generally and demonstrate the central place Hot Springs occupied in the country's broader encounter with syphilis. Placing doctors and health seekers center stage, this book brings medical matters more fully into ongoing discussions on the history of health tourism. At the same time, it also opens a new window onto a crucial period in the history of sexually transmitted diseases.

The "Venereal Peril"

If the period during which Hot Springs earned a reputation as a destination for Americans with syphilis was one of en masse health seeking, it was also one of heightened medical, social, and political interest in VD. Medical authorities at the time believed that syphilis and gonorrhea were "alarmingly on the increase."[50] Though earlier generations had felt their impact, it was only in this era that American physicians began to speak of venereal diseases as a "menace to the national welfare"—as an "evil" that exerted a "degenerating force on the human race."[51] Among the contagions responsible for bringing about "the greatest disasters to society," doctors reported, it was "generally admitted" that there was not one "more serious, more dangerous, or more to be feared than syphilis."[52] More contagious, widespread, and economically destructive than "the dreaded tuberculosis," it was said to be "undoubtedly on the increase," and as venereal specialists documented its "appalling prevalence" all across the United States, the medical profession concluded that syphilis was "a much more common disease than is generally thought."[53] Buttressing their assertions with statistical data, leading authorities on the subject claimed that in conjunction with gonorrhea, roughly one-quarter of the turn-of-the-century American population suffered from some form of venereal disease, while others argued that "from fifty to eighty percent of our people" suffered from these maladies.[54] The upshot of this evidence was clear: Americans were living in an era of great "venereal peril."[55]

Fears of a looming VD epidemic were not confined to the medical profession. As doctors published statistics documenting the extent of venereal infection, social reformers, theologians, political officials, and artists sought to end the "conspiracy of silence" surrounding syphilis and gonorrhea.[56] In 1913, French playwright Eugène Brieux's *Damaged Goods* debuted on Broadway, telling the story of a husband whose premarital sexual escapades later destroyed the health of his wife, their newborn child, and his wife's wet-nurse.[57] In the pages of *Ladies' Home Journal*, Helen Keller expressed outrage at the plight of thousands of newborn boys and girls born blind on account of gonorrheal infections stemming from their fathers' "licentious relations before and since marriage."[58] From the pulpit, religious leaders like Reverend William Lawrence defended efforts to end the "conspiracy of silence" surrounding VD. Acknowledging that editorials like Keller's might "create a panic," Lawrence nevertheless believed that publicizing information about VD was key to reducing "pervasive infection" within the community.[59] "If a panic must be raised," he thundered, "let it come: better panic than defeat or death."[60]

What gave rise to these fears of "death" and "defeat"? Why did diseases once imagined to be entirely private matters suddenly transform into bona fide public health concerns, diseases that authorities regarded as "a menace to the national welfare"? Importantly, the idea that syphilis and gonorrhea were "undoubtedly on the increase" derived less from epidemiology than from other developments—including changes in medical knowledge. Over the course of the nineteenth century, doctors discovered the connections between syphilis and gonorrhea and a whole host of maladies hitherto believed to be entirely unrelated—including infertility, insanity, and ophthalmia neonatorum (a form of infant blindness caused by gonorrhea).[61] On account of these discoveries, diseases once confined to the margins of learned medicine became the object of disciplinary specialization—a phenomenon demonstrated by the appearance of academic titles such as "clinical professor of venereal diseases" and by new publications like the *American Journal of Syphilis* and the *Archives of Dermatology and Syphilology*.[62] By the early twentieth century, doctors had not only discovered syphilis's bacterial cause but had also devised new technologies for diagnosing and treating it.

One of the most important consequences of this venereological research was the recognition of syphilis's chronicity. As doctors today know, syphilis is characterized by three successive phases. In the first, acute stage, infected individuals develop a hard, round, generally painless sore at the site of exposure (usually the penis or vagina). After three to six weeks, this primary lesion disappears, though the infected are still contagious and can transmit syphilis to others through sexual intercourse or (in the case of pregnant women) perinatally to the fetus. If untreated, syphilis then progresses to the secondary stage, which is announced by skin rashes that spread across one or more areas of the body. Other symptoms include fever, sore throat, hair loss, fatigue, frequent head and muscle aches, and weight loss. After this, a period of latency begins that can last for months or years; many patients never progress to the disease's third stage. Those who do experience extensive organ damage, both to the cardiovascular and neurological systems. Tertiary syphilis often leads to dementia, paralysis, ocular impairments, and death. Prior to the discovery of penicillin in the early 1940s, secondary and tertiary syphilis were much more common than they are today.

Knowledge of this prompted doctors to declare that "our hospitals, asylums, madhouses, blind institutions, and epileptic colonies are filled to overflowing with patients who are paying the penalty of syphilis."[63] Informed by the aforementioned discoveries, they began to attribute more and more of the conditions their patients presented to venereal infection, contending that while gonorrhea was responsible for roughly 80 percent of women's pelvic disorders, between 30 to 50 percent of all sterility cases they handled, and fully one-third of all instances of neonatal ophthalmia, syphilis was the root cause of nearly half of all spontaneous abortions and miscarriages, 90 percent of all cases of tabes dorsalis, and the chief etiological factor in about 80 percent of the insanity diagnoses they rendered.[64] Sounding the alarm, one worried practitioner wrote of the perils of living in a society in which "our young women . . . are being mutilated and unsexed by surgical life-saving measures because of these diseases, particularly gonorrhea. Young men are filling our institutions for the defective and insane, because of the ravages of syphilis. Sightless children and grown men and women are crying out in their blindness against this arch crime of gonorrhea; the souls of infants born only to die or to suffer, cry out against the infamy of uncured syphilis."[65] All of this convinced them that "the civilized world is rapidly becoming syphilized."[66] Indeed, numerous physicians testified that a "great Red Plague" was sweeping across the United States.[67]

The idea of a venereal peril, however, did not owe only to improved medical knowledge.[68] When contemporary authorities spoke of syphilis as an "evil" that stalked the land, they did so largely on account of anxieties bred by broader social, economic, and cultural processes.[69] Among these were industrialization, urbanization, and immigration. In the aftermath of the Civil War, the country's economic base rapidly shifted away from agriculture and toward manufacturing, and the resultant industrialization spurred massive demographic change. A highly rural population increasingly gravitated toward urban centers, where native-born white and black Americans (the latter recently delivered from slavery) rubbed shoulders with millions of new arrivals from southern and eastern Europe. With urbanization and immigration came a great deal of labor strife, as unions and business owners violently battled over wages, hours, and workplace conditions. In addition to this, the boom-and-bust cycles of industrial capitalism generated widespread poverty and unemployment—the results of which could be seen in the dilapidated, unsanitary tenements that housed most of urban America's inhabitants. In their day-to-day lives, the working poor contended not only with exploitative employers and landlords but also with deadly diseases such as tuberculosis and regular outbreaks of typhoid fever, typhus, diphtheria, and other infectious maladies. Veritable cesspits of contagion, American cities earned a reputation as the scourge of civilization.

Syphilis was among those diseases most highly associated with urban life. Said to be only rarely encountered in "rural districts," it was something "most extensively met with in large cities," in "the very heart of civilization."[70] Here, the disease spared neither the factory hand nor the aristocrat, neither the "habitué of the slums" nor "those of the higher intellectual sphere."[71] In explaining the connection between syphilis and urban life, authorities revealed some of the social and cultural foundations of the idea of a venereal peril—namely, a fear that the United States, a nation that had long believed itself to be immune to the kinds of economic, demographic, and sociopolitical problems characteristic of European countries, was now experiencing these very problems. Such a realization clashed with Americans' own sense of national identity, as can be seen from the writings of an Oklahoma doctor named Curtis R. Day. In 1912, Day penned an essay arguing that VD was "inseparable from human society in large communities."[72] "Nations have wrestled with the problem," he continued, "only to fail with it." Wherever population increased, "there seems to thrive this monster. It seems in our country, as population again increases, when the frontiers are moving farther away from us until after the frontiers have disappeared and the people have gathered together, it has lifted its hydra head here, and we are now tramping over the same ground and wrestling with the same proposition that the older civilized nations have been struggling with since time began."[73] Emanating from the city, syphilis was "one of the greatest evils of civilization," inspiring near-apocalyptic levels of fear.[74] Indeed, Day was but one of many who regarded syphilis as "one of those terrible destroyers" that stalked the country with "defiant footsteps and increasing power."[75]

For many Americans, the "footsteps" that spread syphilis were those of the prostitute. According to one early twentieth-century estimate, New York City was home to roughly seventy-five thousand prostitutes, and authorities contended that other leading urban centers contained the "same number in proportion to their population[s]."[76] Opinions varied as to the causes of prostitution. For some, the sex trade was a simple reflection of material circumstances—particularly, the "starvation wages" that drove women into "vice" and the "high cost of living" that prevented men from marrying and forming families.[77]

Others saw prostitution as more of a biological phenomenon. Instead of contending that lack of employment or bad family environments forced women into sex work, they argued that there was an "innate tendency" to prostitution.[78] The "lewd" life of the brothel inmate appealed only to those with "depraved taste," a feeble intellect, and a complete "absence of moral sense."[79] Such tendencies were a sign of physical and moral degeneration.[80] Over the course of many centuries, doctors believed, women had developed a sense of morality rooted in "motherly love, limitless self-denial and readiness for sacrifice."[81] Women were thought to be largely asexual and relatively uninterested in carnal matters; it was only in prostitutes, the argument ran, that women's erstwhile "polyandric tendencies" were still evident. As one venereal specialist explained, this owed to "the presence of aberrant cell formations in the brain of primeval origin. A life of vice in women indicates therefore a deeper downfall and a reverting into primitive conditions out of which Nature has elevated her."[82] Such "atavistic abnormalities" as these marked prostitutes as a degenerate, subspecies of women, one completely lacking in intelligence, beauty, education, or refinement.[83]

Regardless of their views as to why it existed, doctors concurred that prostitution was "the fountainhead of gonorrhea and syphilis."[84] Instead of reflecting a straightforward epidemiological reality (one acknowledging the role men play in transmitting infection), the contention that female sex workers were the *"fons et origo* of venereal diseases" largely drew on fears stemming from broader changes in gender relations and women's lived experiences.[85] During the late nineteenth and early twentieth centuries, an increasing number of American women began pursuing higher education, professional careers, and a greater role in public life. Less homebound than the women of previous generations, these "new women" had fewer children than their antebellum predecessors. Some never married at all, and others took advantage of liberalized divorce laws to sever unwanted marital bonds.[86]

For many middle- and upper-class white men, these changes were most un-welcome. Worried by their increasingly public presence in American society, they opposed women's agitation for voting rights, for greater access to postsecondary education, and for a variety of other social and economic freedoms in the same way they opposed prostitution—that is, by claiming that these things violated the role nature had assigned to women through centuries of human evolution. And as this suggests, doctors' fixation on prostitution as the point of origin for all cases of syphilis and gonorrhea followed from their belief that sex work was symptomatic of more general, dissatisfactory transformations in women's lives. Thus, when medical authorities expressed concern over "mutilated and unsexed" female patients, what motivated them was not just the knowledge that syphilis and gonorrhea could damage their reproductive systems, but also a fear that VD might further erode the doctrine of "separate spheres." Similarly, what fostered concern over the patients "filling our institutions of the defective and insane" was not simply a newfound awareness of syphilis's neurological and psychological se-quelae but also a concern that this malady had the potential to accelerate the phenomenon of declining fertility among native-born whites—which sociolo-gists and President Theodore Roosevelt labeled "race suicide".[87] As all of this indicates, fears of a gendered and racialized sort factored highly into the era's "venereal peril."

The notion of a venereal peril was also a product of geopolitical affairs. Among the world's major colonial powers, the late nineteenth and early twentieth centu-ries were a time marked by growing concerns over the stability of imperial structures. With England's near-defeat during the Boer War (1899–1902), Rus-sia's defeat at the hands of the Japanese in 1905, and a number of large-scale up-risings and rebellions threatening colonial rule throughout Africa, the Middle East, and Asia, questions regarding the biological fitness of Western militaries— and by extension, of whites' assumed racial superiority—became a topic of na-tional discussion in many European states. The search for answers often led to VD, especially as medical officers documented rising rates of syphilis and gon-orrhea among colonial militaries.[88] Now imagined as the great toppler of empires, VD became an intense object of concern for Britain, France, and Germany, all of which blamed colonized populations for sapping the fighting strength of their respective armed forces.[89] What followed was a series of incredibly coercive cam-paigns designed to reduce the mobility and control the sexuality of native women, whose bodies were subjected to unparalleled levels of medical surveil-lance and intervention.[90] Though entirely unsuccessful and often subverted, these public health efforts demonstrate the global reach of the "venereal peril" while also drawing attention to the historical process of othering they contributed to.[91]

The same kinds of concerns surfaced with regard to the US military. According to official statistics, in the four decades following the end of the Civil War, rates of syphilis declined within the US military. But with the United States' acquisition of Puerto Rico and the Philippines during the Spanish-American War of 1898, army and navy officials began to fear a reversal of these promising trends. Observing an uptick in the prevalence of VD among European military forces operating in colonial contexts, authorities prepared for similar increases among American soldiers. Their worries were not unfounded. In 1899, the VD admission rate for the US Army increased from 84.5 per 10,000 to 138 per 10,000; by 1900, this had reached 155 per 10,000.[92] By 1902, the US military boasted a rate of venereal sickness higher than that of any imperial power save the United Kingdom.[93] As the United States prepared to enter the First World War in 1917, military doctors reported that VD was "the greatest cause of disability" in the armed services, as rates of syphilis and gonorrhea exceeded those for all other communicable diseases combined.[94] Doctors made similar claims during the Second World War.

The fact that increased concern over sexually transmitted infections mirrored the United States' rise to global power status is not a coincidence. Indeed, the "venereal peril" was in many ways a reaction to the demise of Victorian culture and society. While designed to end the "conspiracy of silence" surrounding syphilis and gonorrhea, the nation's burgeoning venereal discourse was also an attempt on the part of middle- and upper-class white men to maintain their hold on the reins of power at a time in which their privileged position atop the nation's social and political order was under attack.[95] Because syphilis and gonorrhea seemed to hold the key to addressing these preexisting threats, they attracted the interests of doctors, social reformers, and governmental officials all across the country. Absent them, the "venereal peril" would have likely never existed.

The response to VD left no corner of American society untouched. In their attempts to stem the tide of syphilis and gonorrhea, concerned individuals formed groups such as the American Social Hygiene Association, which conducted public awareness campaigns and advocated for the elimination of prostitution. Believing that "virtually all prostitutes carried VD," state governments undertook an aggressive assault on sex work, abolishing red light districts throughout the country and incarcerating thousands of "loose" women—many of whom were *not* prostitutes.[96] In addition to using these legal methods, a number of states passed "eugenic marriage laws" requiring that prospective spouses be declared free from venereal infection before their weddings.[97] In Washington, DC, the federal government passed a law requiring that privately practicing physicians report all cases of VD to local health authorities, while also requiring that medical examiners at Ellis Island and other points of entry inspect all immigrants for VD.[98] In classrooms all across the country, educators played upon fears of venereal infection to instill the idea of premarital sexual abstinence in their students' minds.[99] At the same time, courts began to deregulate the sale and use of condoms, arguing that their value in preventing the spread of VD outweighed moral arguments about their propensity to encourage illicit sex.[100]

The federal government's response to the "venereal peril" culminated in a number of high-profile undertakings, including the Tuskegee Study of Untreated Syphilis in the Negro Male (1932–1972), the Chicago Syphilis Control Project (1937–1940), and the intensive antivenereal campaigns of the First and Second World Wars.[101] The Tuskegee study was overseen and directed by the PHS, which selected 407 syphilitic black men from Macon County, Alabama, and purposefully withheld treatment from them (even after the introduction of penicillin in the early 1940s) in order to test the hypothesis that syphilis "developed differently in blacks and whites."[102] The PHS also participated in the Chicago Syphilis Control Project, a joint venture in which many city and state-wide agencies and organizations (among them the Chicago Medical Society and the Illinois Social Hygiene Board) banded together to promote mass testing and treatment among Chicago residents.[103]

In their analyses of these campaigns, historians have argued that modern American responses to syphilis reflect "a struggle between the moral and biomedical views of disease."[104] As Allan Brandt's classic study has shown, medical authorities disagreed on the optimal means for reducing rates of VD. Throughout the late nineteenth and early twentieth centuries, "Victorian moral norms" clashed with a "new, secular, scientific paradigm."[105] In this battle of "sin vs. science," it was more often the former approach that triumphed, as a belief that syphilis constituted a "punishment for sexual irresponsibility" led the era's antivenereal campaigners to privilege a response to this disease rooted not in medical treatment but in morality—in "repression, continence, and discipline."[106] In aiming to stem the tide of syphilis, authorities practiced the "science of moral engineering," an approach to disease control that led (among other things) to the most aggressive attack on prostitution in the nation's history.[107]

Subsequent scholarship has largely affirmed Brandt's conclusions. In their own studies, historians such as Suzanne Poirier, Lynn Sacco, Marilyn Hegarty, John Parascandola, and Susan Reverby have further explored the ways in which racial and sexual stereotypes, gender biases, and class-based anxieties informed an early twentieth-century approach to VD control in the United States that was driven more by "sin" than "science."[108] As their work reveals, the era's medical authorities targeted not only prostitutes and "promiscuous" women but also blacks, immigrants, homosexuals, the poor, and other socioeconomically marginalized groups. Historical analyses of these coercive and highly repressive state-directed campaigns lend support to Brandt's contention that syphilis in pre-penicillin America was "pre-eminently a disease of the 'other.'"[109]

As this brief review of the historical literature suggests, scholars have painted a compelling and fairly comprehensive portrait of syphilis in pre-penicillin America. Nevertheless, important questions remain to be asked of the early twentieth century's "venereal peril." Perhaps the most interesting of these concern the ways the "wages of sin" interpretation of syphilis shaped the thinking and actions of this malady's victims. How did the era's venereal stigma influence the beliefs and behaviors of the nation's syphilis-stricken men and women? How did venereal sufferers' attempts to deal with this debilitating condition square with the attitudes and prescriptions of those who directed the war against venereal disease? And to what extent did the association between syphilis and sexual immorality govern the ways venereal patients and their doctors diagnosed and treated this disease?

In recent years, scholars have begun to consider these hitherto unexplored matters. Recognizing that in addition to being an ideological prop, syphilis was also a "very real corporeal struggle," they have turned to the history of VD for insights into the changing nature of clinical practice, of doctor-patient relations, and of shifts in the training and education of medical professionals.[110] Collectively, these attempts to tell "a different story of VD" have pushed the boundaries of scholarly debate beyond the historiography's traditional parameters—that is, beyond "morality and the control of women."[111] In stepping outside this "panoptic perspective," historians have come to see that a variety of other factors influenced past generations' responses to syphilis and gonorrhea, including professional, scientific, and practical factors.[112] At the same time, attending to what Anne Hanley terms the "negative space" in VD historiography has afforded a much clearer understanding of how concerns both clinical *and* cultural influenced attempts to diagnose and treat syphilis.[113]

Given its status as a sanctuary for syphilitics, Hot Springs offers an excellent opportunity to further these discussions. Instead of focusing solely on the state and on public health responses to syphilis, this book revolves around therapeutic encounters and questions of medical practice. The value in decentering the state is threefold. First, it opens the stage to privately practicing physicians, patients, and a variety of other local actors typically excluded from historical accounts of VD. Second, it prompts recognition of the fact that syphilis was not only a wartime worry but was also an object of concern during peacetime among civilians lacking any connection to military conflicts. Third, it forces acknowledgment of syphilis's status as both an infectious malady and a chronic condition that impacted the lives of countless men and women year after year, decade after decade.

How might the history of VD appear if we take into account syphilis's complex biological realities and if we assess this subject from the standpoint of doctors and patients and local communities and in the context of peacetime developments? To begin with, this history would demonstrate, as Kevin Sienna has said of early modern England, that syphilis was "a fact of life," something "that touched a much larger portion of the population than we previously imagined, rich and poor, men and women."[114] Those who contracted, suffered from, and transmitted this disease represented a much broader swath of American society than those marginalized groups targeted by the state and included not only rural southern blacks, immigrants, and working-class prostitutes but also white men and women of affluence. As individuals from all of these groups contributed to Hot Springs' health-seeking clientele, comparing their experiences allows for a new, more comprehensive understanding of how race, class, gender, and sexuality informed responses to syphilis in the modern United States.

A second point of contrast with the traditional narrative pertains to syphilis's chronic dimensions. Until the 1940s, this disease was anything but a passing illness, and Americans regularly encountered individuals suffering from secondary and tertiary syphilis. Struggling as they did with locomotor ataxia, tabes dorsalis, insanity, infertility, and other symptoms of secondary and tertiary syphilis, the experiences of Hot Springs' venereal health seekers illustrate the decades-long trail of ailments that often followed in the wake of the disease's contraction. While governments, social reformers, and public health leaders fixated on syphilis's acute, infectious phase, for doctors and the general public, it was the chronic side of this disease that often mattered most. Given this, it behooves us not only to examine particular flashpoints in modern American responses to VD but also to employ a *longue durée* approach and trace out the connections between broader developments (wars, antivenereal campaigns, antiprostitution drives, etc.) and the countless, small-scale, day-to-day interactions between doctors and patients in a variety of clinical settings.[115] Understanding social, political, and medical responses to the "venereal peril," in other words, requires an understanding of how Americans dealt with syphilis's late-stage complications.

A third and final component of the "new narrative" pertains to the relationship between culture and clinical practice. As historians have repeatedly demonstrated, stigma and shame are recurring themes in the history of sexually transmitted infections. Because these have consistently been seen as illnesses contracted by those who violate existing codes of morality, public health responses to syphilis and gonorrhea have been and continue to be highly punitive and discriminatory in nature. But how has this understanding of VD influenced the work of privately practicing physicians? And how exactly has it complicated sufferers' personal and social lives? In order to more fully understand how syphilis is "enmeshed in wider relations of power and inequality," it is critical to examine this disease from a clinical, patient-centered perspective.[116]

With regard to the United States, one recent attempt to look at VD from this vantage point is Lynn Sacco's *Unspeakable: Father-Daughter Incest in American History*. Detailing the medical profession's response to a perceived epidemic of vulvovaginitis among American girls during the late nineteenth and early twentieth centuries, Sacco's analysis reveals how gendered assumptions, attitudes toward sexuality, and racial beliefs shaped the clinical experience. With the discovery of the gonococcus in 1879, doctors recognized that many of the cases of vulvovaginitis they had diagnosed were gonorrheal in origin. This finding immediately prompted them to consider the possibility, Sacco notes, that girls diagnosed with gonorrheal vulvovaginitis were victims of rape by incestuous fathers. Yet only when dealing with "ignorant Italians, Chinese, and Negroes" did doctors conclude as such; when it came to the daughters of socially respectable, "well to do" fathers, most medical practitioners argued that "nonsexual modes of transmission" were responsible.[117] Postulating wildly unscientific ideas, some opined that "a drop of gonorrheal pus on the toilet seat in a public school can start [an] epidemic."[118] The divergent, class-based etiologies doctors built up for this condition, Sacco shows, furthered VD's associations with various "others."[119]

While Sacco's examination draws attention to certain clinical facets of the "venereal peril," it is relatively silent on matters of treatment. What did individuals diagnosed with VD do? According to the conventional wisdom, the "wages of sin" interpretation of syphilis led Americans to conclude that "behavioral and moral means" were the "best way to combat venereal disease."[120] As the description of patients in Hot Springs "working out a case of gonorrheal rheumatism" and "recovering" from a syphilitic spinal lesion suggests, however, people with VD did not necessarily agree with this view. Though syphilis might have secured "victory" over many infected individuals, their deaths should not be read as an indication that resignation and passive acceptance were the primary responses to this disease. Hot Springs, a town in which professional physicians, quack doctors, public health officials, and military surgeons administered many different kinds of treatments to thousands of health seekers between the 1870s and 1940s, suggests otherwise. Therefore, the view that therapeutic approaches to syphilis have remained "secondary" throughout modern American history needs to be reexamined.[121]

In Search of Sexual Health offers such a reexamination. Looking at Hot Springs' history from the standpoint of diagnostic and therapeutic practices, it locates this remote, seemingly isolated central Arkansas locale at the center of the country's broader struggle with syphilis during the late nineteenth and early twentieth centuries. While the existing narrative of venereal disease largely revolves around the actions of governmental and military officials, prominent social reformers, and elite physicians, Hot Springs shows that responses to syphilis were often shaped by a variety of *nonstate actors* as well, whose interests, circumstances, and behaviors influenced clinical decisions around this disease to a much greater extent than hitherto acknowledged. Hot Springs' salience can also be seen in the way the city mediated conflicts within American medicine at this time: between "moral" and "medical" responses to syphilis, traditional and modern methods of venereological diagnosis and treatment, and reductionist and holistic public health strategies, as well as debates over the role of race, class, gender, and sexuality in treatment paradigms and procedures. Within Hot Springs, the working out of these conflicts consistently yielded policies and practices reflecting the interests of local people—whether resident doctors, visiting patients, or permanent residents. The city's history thus offers a new narrative of a crucial era in the United States' struggle with sexually transmitted illness.

Outline of the Book

What social, cultural, and economic forces and factors conspired to make Hot Springs the destination of choice for venereal health seekers? Addressing this question, chapter 1 examines the health resort's formative years through the eyes of Archie Cowles, a Cleveland native who in 1907 traveled there in order to be treated for syphilis. As his experiences show, while the disease's status as the "wages of sin" underwrote Hot Springs' transformation into a harbor for those with syphilis, its stigmatized status exerted less influence over the day-to-day lives of the city's health seekers than might be expected. Instead of withdrawing from the world on account of internalized feelings of shame and guilt, many visiting syphilitics eagerly sought out bodily cures for their ailments and forged close bonds of friendship and camaraderie with fellow patients. Within the destigmatized social environment they built within the city, moralistic assessments of VD ceded ground to more materialistic, socioeconomic etiologies. Cowles's patient narrative thus complicates the "sin vs. science" framework that has governed historical analyses of sexually transmitted illness. Though often presented as an ideological battle between morality and medicine, the "venereal peril" emerges as more complex when one examines it from the standpoint of clinical practice.

This is not to suggest that morality played no role in Hot Springs' response to syphilis. As chapter 2 makes clear, turn-of-the-century resort doctors believed that absent the correction of those immoral and ungodly habits imagined as syphilis's root cause, this venereal disease would remain incurable. In light of this belief, they crafted a form of antivenereal therapy that combined drugs like mercury, the city's near-boiling waters, and a series of behavioral measures referred to as "moral treatment." In simultaneously aiming to heal body, mind, and soul, local medical practitioners seamlessly merged approaches to VD that historians have typically interpreted as polar opposites. Based on the published writings of the city's physicians and the correspondence of a syphilitic patient named Michael J. Murphy, this chapter draws attention to how religious and scientific views on venereal disease often intersected, cooperated, and reinforced each other. Within Hot Springs, the boundaries between "science" and "sin" were often incredibly porous.

In many ways, this hybridized medico-moral system of antivenereal therapy was the product of highly local concerns. Concerned that medicine's professional elite viewed their practices in an unfavorable light simply because they deigned to treat the venereally afflicted, local physicians approached syphilis from a behavioral standpoint in part so as to demonstrate their own moral rectitude. Moreover, inculcating a sense of shame and guilt in the minds of their predominantly white clientele served an important ideological function, as it carved a color line through a disease that, especially in the South, was heavily associated with "amoral" African Americans. "Hygienic treatment" thus demonstrates the impact of postbellum racial anxieties on turn-of-the-century understandings of and approaches to VD.

Hot Springs' response to syphilis maintained its unique, local nature into the early twentieth century. The period between the 1910s and 1930s witnessed both the introduction of new, laboratory-derived methods for diagnosing and treating syphilis *and* the federal government's mounting of a public health campaign designed to eradicate the "venereal peril" from American society. One of the first of the early twentieth century's venereal innovations to impact Hot Springs was the Wassermann test, an advanced, syphilis-detecting procedure invented in 1905 by the German scientist August Wassermann. Looking at the impact this medical technology had on local doctors' knowledge of and experiences with syphilis, chapter 3 turns to the Army and Navy General Hospital, a Hot Springs–based military infirmary that between the 1890s and 1910s cared for hundreds of syphilis-stricken soldiers and sailors. Shortly after the Wassermann's introduction, resident surgeons' understanding of syphilis underwent a dramatic transformation, as a disease once not well understood at all now became a malady whose boundaries were clearly demarcated and whose accurate diagnosis proved a much less trying affair than it had previously been. Yet while laboratory science definitely played a role in doctors' new understanding of syphilis, what proved crucial at Army and Navy was the hospital's admissions policy, which until 1910 barred (officially, at least) the entrance of venereally afflicted servicemen. Before this time, a fear of detection and denial of medical services had led prospective patients to hide and conceal any evidence of a past or present syphilitic infection, but the lifting of the ban made deception unnecessary and so enabled doctors to gather the kinds of open and honest case histories believed essential to the accurate diagnosis of syphilis. Thus, even after laboratory science's arrival in Hot Springs, it was a rather traditional source of diagnostic insight—patient testimony—that informed how local physicians understood syphilis.

The fact that so many Army and Navy patients freely divulged the secrets of their sex lives to doctors suggests that early twentieth-century responses to syphilis were not solely moralistic. The evidence from the Hot Springs VD clinic, a federally run medical center that between 1921 and 1936 provided free treatment to over sixty thousand patients—black as well as white, male as well as female—indicates that its response was likewise not primarily driven by morality. During the first few years of its existence, the PHS officials in charge of the clinic conducted a rather conventional antivenereal campaign, emphasizing personal responsibility, cracking down on prostitution, and utilizing modern laboratory technologies such as Salvarsan (an arsenical compound invented in 1910) and the Wassermann test. However, as chapter 4 reveals, this initial focus on behavioral, legal, and scientific approaches to syphilis rather quickly gave way to more environmentally rooted disease control work, as patients' desperate material circumstances demonstrated to clinic personnel that America's venereal problems were a matter not just of morals, germs, and drugs but also of food, shelter, and money. Acknowledging that *poverty* was the central impediment to syphilis's eradication, the PHS pivoted toward a series of extramedical measures designed to ensure that patients remained in Hot Springs long enough to complete the required course of treatment.

While these policies benefited all of the clinic's patients, they did not do so in an equitable fashion. Throughout the 1920s and 1930s, the PHS consistently set the needs of white health seekers above those of black syphilitics. Driven by a eugenic desire to practice "race conservation," clinic director Oliver Wenger provided extra levels of support (in both an informal and institutional sense) to the white men and women who entered his facility.[122] White men were particularly singled out for governmental largesse, as during the Great Depression the PHS operated a transient center (named Camp Garraday) solely for the clinic's white male patients, who received food, shelter, and domiciliary care and were given opportunities for work and recreation while undergoing treatment. None of these generous provisions were offered to African American men and women, who faced considerable hostility and discrimination (from both local residents and clinic personnel) in Hot Springs, experienced lower levels of care, and left the city with worse health outcomes. Shedding new light on the racialized nature of early twentieth-century public health policy, this chapter in the city's history also provides a deeper context for understanding other aspects of the government's response to syphilis—including the Tuskegee study.

As PHS officials knew quite well, the existence of the Hot Springs VD clinic threatened to displace private practitioners from the city's medical marketplace. So too did the introduction of more powerful medical technologies such as the Wassermann test and Salvarsan. During the next two decades, a number of well-established physicians saw their businesses shrink, and as chapter 5 shows, in response to these challenges, local doctors drastically modified their approach to syphilis. Abandoning "hygienic" remedies, resort healers increasingly began offering purely hydrotherapeutic forms of antivenereal care. In defense of this approach, they advanced two central claims: that "water cure" was a time-honored system of therapy, one whose efficacy had been demonstrated by ancient healers such as Hippocrates, and that the springs' ability to cure syphilis was a product of their *radioactivity*, something revealed by chemical analyses of the city's waters. Such arguments resonated with the increasingly *holistic* nature of medical practice during the interwar period, an era in which increasing numbers of physicians on both sides of the Atlantic criticized modern laboratory methods and proposed a variety of antireductionist alternatives designed to augment the body's natural healing powers. By tapping into these developments, the healers of Hot Springs realized a means of preserving their medical livelihoods as venereal specialists.

Moreover, the evidence from Hot Springs challenges the claims of existing studies of American medical holism in that it indicates that this movement was impelled by both clinical and cultural concerns. With regard to the latter, the shift from hygiene to hydrotherapy signaled contemporary fears of "overcivilization"— that is, the idea that American men had become weak, effeminate, and overly refined with the growth of consumer capitalism. As a therapeutic system, water cure took aim at these ailments, seeking to heal the syphilitic body by placing patients in contact with the "barbarian virtues" of primitive and premodern medical cultures. Thus, even as the role of morality in Hot Springs steadily declined during the 1920s and 1930s, the city's response to syphilis remained closely tied to broader matters of race, class, and gender.

As this brief overview indicates, Hot Springs' response to syphilis changed considerably over the course of the late nineteenth and early twentieth centuries. In part, the city's shifting therapeutic culture reflected changes in the demographic status of Hot Springs' venereal clientele, as with the passage of time a place initially existing as a watering hole for the well-to-do (i.e., white middle- and upper-class males) became by the 1920s and 1930s largely a preserve of the indigent. At the same time, these changes followed on developments of a medico-scientific and technological sort, as the venereological advances of the twentieth century's first decade brought into resident healers' disease-fighting armamentarium a variety of new tools for understanding, diagnosing, and treating syphilis—among them the Wassermann test and Salvarsan. As these developments demonstrate, Hot Springs was neither isolated from nor immune to the broader changes that swept through American medicine and society between the 1890s and 1930s. Despite this, however, the city's response to syphilis was consistently shaped by local forces and factors.

Hot Springs presents a number of new questions about America's experience with syphilis, questions that force us to consider anew the nation's venereal past. That in Hot Springs this disease often affected white men of means; that its progress through the body often left victims with chronic impairments of cerebral and nervous function; that those who suffered under it often devised their own means for dealing with their conditions—all of this suggests that there is much more to say about the history of the United States' venereal struggles, that there exists another side to the story of this nation's response to syphilis in the period prior to penicillin. Indeed, from this study of Hot Springs emerges a different understanding of the late nineteenth and early twentieth centuries' great "venereal peril," one whose historical importance extends beyond this single southern city, providing insight into the broader, nationwide contours of America's battles with VD.

CHAPTER ONE

The Emergence of Hot Springs as a Haven for the American Syphilitic, 1880–1910

Archie Cowles was a sick man; that much was clear. Between April 1906 and May 1907, Cowles's health steadily deteriorated, as an "aching swollen throat," a "dull headache," "perpetual fatigue," and "distressed breathing" rendered him unfit for work and unable to enjoy the company of friends and family. On top of these symptoms, Cowles suffered from progressive loss of hearing and found his voice "so husky I can scarcely make myself understood." "I am in bad shape," he confided to a cousin at one point; "words cannot tell how I suffer." So distressed was he that on one occasion Cowles contemplated an impending trip "across the Great Divide into the Unknown."[1]

Instead of acting on these gloomy ruminations, however, Cowles opted to fight his illness. In early July 1907, Cowles left his hometown of Cleveland for Hot Springs, Arkansas. After a few days of railway travel, he reached the place whose far-famed waters had helped transform this remote central Arkansas town into one of the country's premier health resorts. Indeed, Cowles found that at the resort he was but one of hundreds of men and women who had crossed the country in the hopes of curing an "incurable" sickness that he attributed, as he wrote on October 1, 1907, to "the bitterness of the prostitute": syphilis. Through their collective acts of health seeking, Hot Springs became a sanctuary for syphilitics in America. How and why did this happen, and what kinds of experiences did Cowles and his fellow syphilitics meet with in Hot Springs?

In addressing these questions, this chapter opens a window onto a relatively unexplored side of the United States' turn-of-the-century encounter with syphilis. While historians have examined its social construction as a stigmatized disease of "the other," little is known about how that stigma influenced the lives of people with VD. What meanings did sufferers attribute to their syphilitic illnesses? What curative strategies did they employ in the attempt to restore

health? Traditionally, historians have argued that because of the widespread belief that syphilis and gonorrhea constituted a form of punishment for sexual sin,
therapeutic responses to VD were "secondary" to behavioral and moralistic ones.[2]
According to this interpretation, the view that syphilis was the "wages of sin" bred
a "conspiracy of silence" around the disease, one that encouraged sufferers to pas-
sively accept their illnesses and stymied the development of *medical* solutions to
VD—which, accordingly, quickly reached epidemic proportions.[3]

Hot Springs offers a different, more complex narrative of the late nineteenth-
and early twentieth-century "venereal peril." It shows that while the era's stigmatized perceptions of VD forcefully impacted the lives of people with syphilis,
they neither reduced them to states of inaction nor foreclosed the pursuit of curative therapies. As moralistic understandings of syphilis pushed the infected
away from local sources of medical care, they also pulled them toward Hot
Springs—a place said to have been created by a benevolent, forgiving God who
promised health to the wayward. A product of the "wages of sin" mentality, Hot
Springs attracted venereal health seekers in need of cures that were simultaneously directed at mind, body, and spirit. Like Archie Cowles, most of the city's
VD patients were white men, who, for cultural, social, and economic reasons,
found travel to Hot Springs easier than did nonwhites and women. As this suggests, realities of race, gender, and class shaped Hot Springs' transformation into
a haven for American syphilitics.

Instead of silencing discussion of venereal illness and curtailing the development of medical responses to it, then, the language of shame surrounding
syphilis stimulated new discourses and led to the creation of novel forms of therapeutic behavior. Yet Hot Springs' response to syphilis was about more than
morality. Though it drove individuals like Archie Cowles to the city, syphilis's
sinful status did not universally govern the conduct of the venereally afflicted. As
visitors familiarized themselves with other health seekers, the "wages of sin" narrative ceded ground to new etiological theories rooted in ideas about economic
hardship and intolerance. With the passage of time, a relatively destigmatized
environment emerged in Hot Springs, and this laid the groundwork for alternative conceptions of VD.

The Benefit of the Baths

As spring turned to autumn and then winter, Archie Cowles continued to worsen.
By the spring of 1907, he had had enough. "These N.E. winds are killing me by
inches" he confided to a friend in a letter dated May 7, 1907. "There is no hope
that I shall survive another winter in the north." Cleveland's "beastly northern

winters" were a recurring problem, bringing a "bad cough" that threatened to drag Cowles's symptoms from his throat down into his "bronchial tubes," as he wrote on June 4, 1907. In the previous year, a friend had seen firsthand how the winter had "taken all [his] strength" and so offered Cowles lodging in his own home, which Cowles politely declined in a May 10, 1906 letter. Cowles instead began to contemplate a trip to Hot Springs.[4] An immediate concern was money. Cowles had made a previous trip to Hot Springs, residing there from December 1905 to April 1906, and in a letter dated December 10, 1905, he complained that "the cheapest a respectable person can live here is $4.20 to $4.50 [per week]." Returning with all his savings depleted, he then took an "insecure" job whose earnings allowed him no more than an "old hovel" as a dwelling place. In his letter of May 10, 1906, Cowles explained to his that he lacked the resources to finance even a short stay in central Arkansas. "Supposing I went broke there," he continued, "and had to go into the swamps in the heat of summer. I should die of malaria. . . . [I]f I have to die I prefer to die in dear old Cleveland rather than in the Arkansas swamps."

Despite his fears of "becom[ing] a vagabond," Archie Cowles ultimately decided to embark for Hot Springs. In June 1907, he secured his father's financial assistance, which a number of friends supplemented through personal monetary donations.[5] Though an "object of charity," Cowles wrote on June 20 that he now had the means to leave his native city. Predicting that "the country air and water will brace me up some," he arrived in Hot Springs—"tired and sick"—just before midnight on July 8, 1907. After securing a room, he enjoyed a quiet, peaceful sleep, and then arose the next morning and began "drinking a lot of lovely hot water." "Awful hot weather," he wrote his parents, adding "love to all."

Cowles took quite well to the local climate, which enabled him to spend a fair amount of time "reading, writing, and sleeping" in the "fine" air of the Ozark Mountains, as he wrote in his July 8 letter. "I fill up with hot water and climb the mountain," he said of a typical day in Hot Springs, noting in a July 31 letter that his "nose and throat [were] better" because of Hot Springs' natural health-giving qualities. In addition to imbibing the local waters, Cowles also made it a daily practice to bathe in them, as he described in a July 14 letter. Early each morning, he walked to a local bathhouse, had his "ticket punched at the desk," then headed

to the clothes room where I undress and hang my clothes in one of the many cupboards. My valuables—watch, keys, money, ticket, etc.—I put in one of my shoes, which I can carry with me to the bathroom. . . . Well, I take my towel and cup and shoe and go through the cooling room into the bathroom. . . . The hot water is hotter than ever now, as it does not cool so much in the pipes, and the 'cold' water is not very cold. . . . One's body is at such a high temperature [in] this weather that he cannot stay in the hot water as long as in the winter. If he stays 20 minutes he does well. Then he begins to feel he must get out, and if he stays in, he will become faint and dizzy. . . . When I get out of the tub I drink 3 or 4 cupfulls of hot water and begin to sweat profusely. . . . Then I drink more hot water and lie down and try to sleep. But I can't sleep because the sweat trickles as it bursts forth and runs away in little streams. Every few minutes I occasionally get into the tub long enough to heat up my skin. When I think I have sweat enough for one day I stop drinking and lie for a long time, till the beads no longer come out on my arms. Then I go to the cooling room and sit till visible perspiration has ceased and I feel cool. Then I go and dress. Usually take a nap after I get home from the bath.

Cowles reported on June 20 that his daily trips to the bathhouses of Hot Springs left him feeling "stronger" and on July 31 that they were improving his health "to a considerable extent." These comments echoed those from a letter Cowles wrote on February 4, 1906, during his first trip to Hot Springs, in which he observed that "as soon drank," the city's waters begin "flowing out of the pores of one's skin, washing out the poisons."

Consistent as it was with contemporary beliefs about the relationship between health and place, Cowles's decision to travel to Hot Springs in search of a cure for syphilis likely did not surprise either friends or family. The city's history as health resort dates back to 1832, when Congress declared that the location (whose waters are continually warmed by heat escaping from the Earth's interior through the myriad fractures and fissures created during the formation of the Ouachita mountains some five hundred million years ago) was to be forever set aside for the "benefit and enjoyment" of the general public.[6] Throughout the antebellum period, word of the springs' therapeutic powers slowly spread across the country, and while men and women suffering from rheumatism, paralysis, neuralgia, and dyspepsia regularly traveled there seeking medical relief, from the 1860s onward, Hot Springs became a particularly popular destination for those afflicted with syphilis. Mid-nineteenth-century doctors who visited the area noted that there were "more old syphilitic cases than any other form of disease that find their way here" and regularly remarked on how the springs had "no rival in the cure of this affliction."[7] Recognizing its growing prominence, in 1877, Congress created the Hot Springs Reservation (HSR). Initially consisting of 2,529 acres, the HSR was public land managed by a federally appointed commission, whose task was to maintain and control access to the 826,000 gallons of water that daily coursed through the site.[8]

If Cowles's decision to journey to Hot Springs would have made sense to contemporaries, his fears of dying of malaria in the "Arkansas swamps" indicate that this was not something undertaken lightly. In fact, Cowles was far from alone in the reservations he expressed about the wisdom of traveling to this part of the country. Throughout the nineteenth century, popular and professional opinion held that white bodies were ill suited for life outside temperate zones. Successful migration to the south, a dangerously hot region with a "tropical" climate, was thought to require a lengthy process of acclimatization (often referred to as "seasoning").[9] Many were unwilling to undergo this in a place regarded as a "hotbed of malaria," which hindered the development of local communities and health resorts all across the South.[10]

Arkansas was just one of many southern locales perceived to be "plague-stricken."[11] Early nineteenth-century accounts of life there reveal widespread fears of "dangerous southern heat," and are replete with denunciations of the various agues and fevers thought to emanate from its "thick, oozing swamps."[12] While usually leveled at low-lying areas in the eastern part of the state, these charges can also be seen in descriptions of the Ozark Mountains of central and northwestern Arkansas. Traveling through Hot Springs in the 1830s, the St. Louis physician George Engelmann observed an "unbearable" summer heat that caused chills and fevers to "rage" all throughout the area. Engelmann also recorded instances of medical visitors being "overpower[ed]" by the springs, as many "fell down in exhaustion and in feverlike sicknesses."[13] A few years later, the medical geographer W. J. Goulding reported on fevers of "very unusual severity and prevalence" in central Arkansas.[14] In the 1870s, a climatological survey of the region boasted that Hot Springs possessed "more advantages for health" than any location of similar latitude, but it nevertheless remained the case that the journey into the resort sometimes brought one through "valleys and swamps . . . that are miasmatic in themselves and unhealthy to a degree."[15] Only gradually did malaria recede from the state; as late as 1901, the president of the Hot Springs Medical Association confided to visiting colleagues that at times, winds from the Arkansas lowlands blew the deadly mosquito "into our midst to ply his nefarious work."[16]

Given their location in a state saddled with an unhealthful reputation, those hoping to transform Hot Springs into a health resort of nationwide renown faced a difficult task. Whereas the western reaches of the country were imagined to be full of salubrious settings, some writers held that southern states were "of little value" in a therapeutic sense.[17] Looking to assuage the concerns raised by prospective health seekers such as Archie Cowles, local physicians stressed that while removed from the "severities of the North," Hot Springs was "not sufficiently far South to make the danger of malaria felt."[18] Epidemics of cholera or yellow fever were also said to be "unknown" there, as the atmosphere of the Ozarks was deemed "to antagonize the invasion of these diseases."[19] And in addition to celebrating the "exceptionally healthy" qualities of the mountainous districts near Hot Springs, resident physicians described cases of syphilis that improved markedly after change from a "very cold" northern climate to the "warm and agreeable" climate of central Arkansas.[20]

This was but one form of civic boosterism used to enhance Hot Springs' popularity. In order to promote travel to the region, enterprising bathhouse owners distributed pamphlets and guidebooks all across the country and placed advertisements in the pages of popular and professional magazines celebrating the springs' life-saving powers.[21] On a more direct, personal level, they also employed business agents known as "drummers," as Cowles noted in his July 14, 1907, letter, to ride the railways in and out of the city in search of prospective patients. Resident physicians sometimes joined in these efforts while also taking advantage of regional and national medical conferences to inform colleagues of their city's miraculous waters—and to invite them to Hot Springs to witness these effects firsthand.[22] Local patent medicine manufacturers drew attention to the region by publishing advertisements for their products in newspapers and journals.[23] And because the city was itself federal property, government officials also took an interest in marketing the region's salubrious qualities, recording testimonials from patients and reprinting these in a variety of different media.[24]

Eventually, word of the "very effective" treatment syphilis met with in Hot Springs found its way not only into medical journals but also into more widely

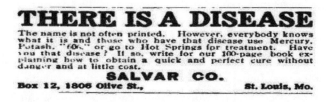

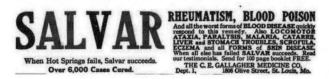

These advertisements for Salvar appeared in *Brotherhood of Locomotive Fireman and Engineers' Magazine* 51 (1911): 736, and *Locomotive Engineers' Journal* 47 (1913): 1151.

circulated weeklies like the *Chautauquan* and popular atlases like *King's Hand-book of the United States*, which spoke of how Hot Springs' waters were "benefi-cial in cases of diseases of the skin . . . and for rheumatism and syphilis."[25] By the late nineteenth century the connection between Hot Springs' waters and the cure of syphilis had been cemented in the public mind. During the 1880s and 1890s, physicians from all across the country spoke of syphilitic patients who had got-ten the "Hot Springs craze" into their heads, while venereal specialists remarked on how the city had "of late become very popular" on account of the widespread belief that its waters "have the power to drive out syphilis completely."[26] As one Kansas City physician put it after traveling to the resort, the number of syphilit-ics in Hot Springs was "almost exhaustless."[27]

Of course, some prospective health seekers were unwilling or unable to at-tempt the journey to the city. While the campaign to combat the notion that Arkansas was nothing more than a "low-lying, swampy country[,] . . . breathing forth malarial poisons," likely convinced some skeptics to travel to the state, others simply could not contemplate this.[28] The popularity of Eureka Springs, a health resort in the northwestern corner of Arkansas, for one, was "handicapped" by what one observer termed "the prevalent misconception of 'worthlessness' that attaches to Arkansas or its products."[29] There were also those who found Hot Springs less than ideal. In 1911, for example, a disgruntled health seeker pro-claimed that though "Hot Springs does not look sick," the "surprising changes of weather" often seen there had a way of negating the resort's therapeutic capabilities.[30]

In addition to those unwilling to hazard a trip to the Ozarks, there were others who faced financial barriers to entry. As the resort's reputation grew, a process of gentrification set in. For much of the nineteenth century, those health-seekers who sojourned at the springs occupied the lower rungs of the country's economic ladder, as the city annually swelled with a "large population" of "poor, miserable paupers."[31] "Nothing but miserable board shanties to be seen anywhere," said an observer of the city after an 1881 trip to the region, noting that one daily met in Hot Springs the "victims of the worst forms of cutaneous diseases, all being here with the hope of getting cured, yet few having money to pay their physicians."[32]

By this time, however, Hot Springs was "fast becoming a fashionable resort."[33] Leasing land and water from the HSR, local developers began replacing the city's "miserable board shanties" with "palatial hotels."[34] Before long, the city had be-come a place of elegance and opulence, a fin-de-siècle paradise whose luxurious accommodations included hotels boasting porcelain tubs and long-distance tele-phones, parks replete with horseback and bicycle paths, tennis courts, and golf courses, and numerous other places of amusement, including an amphitheater where "high-class orchestras" could be heard giving thrice-daily concerts.[35] Bathhouses became increasingly elaborate, updated with state-of-the-art hydrotherapeutic gadgetry such as vapor cabinets, electrical massage, and needle showers. The most lucrative of these was the Fordyce, which local newspapers dubbed "the best equipped bathing establishment in the world."[36] One of its competitors, the Maurice Bathhouse, boasted three-hundred dressing rooms, extra-large tubs, and personalized vapor, shower, and douche rooms. After bathing, guests at the Maurice had the option of continuing on into a sun parlor, a gymnasium, or a private room for relaxation and refreshment. With the passage of time, these kinds of amenities became standard fare along Bathhouse Row.[37]

To ensure that its visitors remained a "people of leisure, with an abundance of money to spend," local officials forcibly uprooted the city's poorer health seekers—those living in "shanties or tents" or found "encamped under the trees with no other shelter."[38] The process of forced removal began in 1877, when General Benjamin F. Kelley, the first superintendent of the Hot Springs Reservation, tore down a popular hillside bathing site for poor syphilitics known as the Ral Hole. Kelley's actions followed on complaints from bathhouse owners who believed that the presence of indigent health seekers in and around Hot Springs was polluting the resort's waters and driving away "thousands" of prospective clients.[39] So as to mollify the inhabitants of the Ral Hole, Kelley obtained federal funding for the construction of a free, government-run bathhouse.[40] Yet this did nothing to counteract local policies aimed at forcing poor health seekers off of resort grounds. In 1901, a visitor reported on how "it was the policy of the municipality of Hot Springs to discourage the coming of the poor people to that place," which it did "by withholding all of the usual eleemosynary institutions from their use."[41] Making matters worse, in 1911, Congress passed a law demanding that all health seekers seeking admission to the government bathhouse swear an oath of destitution; those found to have lied about their impoverished status faced a $25 fine or six days in jail. The next year, the number of baths given at this facility declined by sixty-three thousand.[42]

As a result of its Gilded Age makeover, Hot Springs' clientele diversified: earlier the preserve of the poor, it was increasingly visited by "very wealthy people from the Northern states."[43] By the first decade of the twentieth century, "more than fifty percent" of the city's health seekers were said to be "people of leisure, with an abundance of money to spend, who are in no way the victims of disease other than that of over-work, over-feeding, and conditions brought about by luxurious living."[44] Medical authorities in other locales came to believe that "only the rich" could afford the "costly excursion" to Hot Springs.[45] As a Chicago physician said of his city's syphilitic patients: "Our rich people go to the great Mecca of medical wisdom, to Hot Springs," while "our poor people may go to—where they please."[46]

The idea that "all syphilitics go to Hot Springs," then, was quite simplistic. While syphilis struck rich and poor, black and white, and male and female, individuals from Archie Cowles's demographic predominated within Hot Springs. Women were particularly underrepresented among the city's venereal health seekers, and their comparative absence within Hot Springs illustrates another way the era's venereal stigma influenced the city's transformation into an asylum for syphilitics.

Women, Syphilis, and the Springs

Travel to Hot Springs was a highly gendered phenomenon. According to one resort doctor, while two-fifths of the men who came to Hot Springs were syphilitic, such a disease was seen in "not more than one in twenty among the female invalids."[47] Why was this? What explains the relative absence of venereally infected women at Hot Springs?

One possibility is that women had limited knowledge of VD. According to doctors, the average female syphilitic was entirely "ignorant of the nature of her disease."[48] Explaining this, they emphasized how women's "sensitive modesty" made them "shrink from being examined for syphilis"; as one writer put it, women were often "debarred by feelings of delicacy from discussing the situation as freely as men."[49] While perhaps true in some cases, these statements disguise the fact that in their day-to-day lives, doctors often strove to keep women in a state of venereological ignorance. One way of doing so was to conspire with men known to have infected their wives with syphilis or gonorrhea—a practice known as the "medical secret."

Fearing the domestic upheaval women's knowledge of their venereal infections might bring, husbands sometimes sought "every possible means" of preventing spouses from learning the true nature of their ailments.[50] This included making agreements with doctors, who promised not to inform women about the venereal origins of their illnesses. As one physician put it, "A good woman trusting her husband may go through a long and serious attack of syphilis without ever suspecting what is the matter with her."[51] Speaking in more detail about the "medical secret," a colleague revealed how "over and over again, for the sake of family peace, and perhaps for the sake of the patient herself, we, as medical advisors, are obliged to maintain this state of innocence and ignorance during, it may be, a very long course of treatment. . . . Much still remains to be accomplished before secrecy, that bane to proper treatment in women, can be consigned to the limbo of the past."[52] As this suggests, though some abhorred it, medical men were largely faithful to the demands of the medical secret. So regular was the practice that doctors created a new diagnostic category—"syphilis of the ignorant"—to help them understand how "so much syphilis in married women is unsuspected."[53]

Was this truly the case? While some women may have been ignorant, a number of cases suggest that many women adequately understood the etiology, symptoms, and therapeutics of syphilis.[54] As one local writer had it, the city boasted of many "women broken down in health . . . from the effects of sacrificing at the altar of Venus." One such was Mary Koehler, a Hot Springs native who in 1916 filed for divorce from her husband, a mail carrier named Robert. Over the course of their trial, Mary summoned numerous witnesses who testified as to her husband's physically and verbally abusive behavior. Contesting these allegations, Robert charged that it was his wife who was in the wrong. In defense of this, he called forth "several physicians" who revealed that they had treated Mary for syphilis, and that "she had it for eleven years or more." According to these doctors, prior to their marriage, Mrs. Koehler had informed Robert "she had some female ailment," all the while "conceal[ing] from him" the fact of her tertiary syphilis. During cross-examination, however, the court learned that Robert had "talked" with local doctors in Hot Springs, and that he "knew what was being done" in connection with his wife's condition. This disproved Robert's claims—both that he was ignorant of the true nature of his wife's condition and that she had concealed knowledge of this from him. Her husband's contentions undermined, Mary Koehler was then granted her request for divorce.[55]

This was also true for Margaret Wilson, an Arkansas woman who went before the state's Supreme Court in 1911 requesting a divorce from her husband. Responding to her complaints of abuse and negligence, Wilson's husband averred that shortly after their marriage, Margaret had contracted syphilis and that he had sent her to Hot Springs in order to take "the mercury rubbing treatment and baths." Wilson repudiated these charges and produced testimony from doctors who had "failed to notice any evidence of venereal disease" when treating her for "barrenness." Such a revelation led the presiding judge to grant Mrs. Wilson her wish, and she successfully severed her marital ties to this noted "man of means."[56]

Another woman with a fairly developed understanding of VD was Edna Wade. In 1920, Wade, a native of Kansas City, faced a divorce suit from her husband, who alleged "habitual drunkenness" and "gross misconduct" on her part.

Responding with a countersuit, Wade charged her husband with "cruel treatment," citing a "lump on his neck" that he treated with "mercurial ointment" as evidence of a syphilitic infection. In addition to this, Wade informed the court that her husband "went to Hot Springs nearly every February." Unfortunately for her, this evidence failed to sway the courts. Nevertheless, Wade's testimony indicates that the "medical secret" was not always successful in ensuring women's ignorance of sexually transmitted diseases.[57]

Such a finding squares with recent research documenting how prominently VD figured in women's attempts to combat sexual double standards and the patriarchal institutions that upheld them. Within the emerging genre of "New Woman" fiction, for example, authors such as Sarah Grand used syphilis to condemn male sexual license and to present male bodies as sites of venereal contamination.[58] Inside courtrooms, women used the era's new venereological insights to bolster divorce suits, presenting their own syphilitic or gonorrheal infections as evidence of husbands' adulterous conduct.[59] Operating in a more public manner, women's rights activists identified the "venereal peril" as an indication of men's moral failure—as the inevitable consequence of a society predicated on men's oppression of women.[60] Taken together, these varied actions promoted recognition of women's status as *sufferers* (as opposed to mere transmitters) of VD, while also convincing many doctors and political officials that syphilis and gonorrhea needed to be dealt with in an open, honest manner.

While these cases indicate that turn-of-the-century American women's knowledge of VD ran deeper than previously believed, they also draw attention to some of the reasons that comparatively few female syphilitics journeyed to Hot Springs. For one, as residents of Arkansas, Koehler and Wilson's expenses were minimal; turn-of-the-century women from other parts of the country, in contrast, would have had to raise funds for travel and lodging in Hot Springs, something many would have been hard pressed to do. Secondly, as Arkansas natives, the two women likely faced relatively little danger from traveling (either alone or accompanied) to a place peopled by the sexually "immoral." As historians have repeatedly observed, women with VD faced consequences far more severe than those their male counterparts met with.[61] At a time when campaigns against brothels and prostitutes (whom most assumed to be the chief spreaders of infection) raged across the country, how many female syphilitics in New York, Chicago, or California would have risked public disclosure of their illness while en route to Hot Springs—especially when this could lead to complete loss of social status and reputation?[62] Undoubtedly, these gendered realities factored into women's relative absence in Hot Springs. As one observer noted, the disease's association with immorality meant that Hot Springs "[could not] be very pleasant to ladies of refinement."[63]

Clearly, the "benefit of the baths" was not open to any and all venereal patients. On account of economic, racial, and gendered factors, women were much less likely to do what Archie Cowles did in the summer of 1907. For the most part, the kinds of individuals who transformed the region into sanctuary for syphilitics were, like Cowles, white males possessed of some wealth. How did their health-seeking behaviors align with the era's prevailing ideas about syphilis?

The Wages of Sin

As hundreds of individuals like Archie Cowles began traveling to Hot Springs and kindred sites in search of cures for syphilis, contemporary venereologists were forced to grapple with the "popularity of these resorts."[64] What explains the emergence of this remarkable form of therapeutic behavior? Scholarly examinations of contemporary health tourism often cite financial considerations as a prime reason for medical travel, noting that those who engage in this do so because the sought-after treatment or procedure is less costly abroad than it would be in their own country. Available historical evidence suggests that its nineteenth- and twentieth-century analogue also "operated within the context of economic relations."[65] Given his fears of "becoming a vagabond," this was certainly the case for Archie Cowles. But practical concerns alone did not induce syphilitics to seek therapeutic treatment. Social and cultural factors played a role as well. With re-gard to sexually transmitted diseases, decisions about therapeutic behavior were made in an environment powerfully shaped by syphilis's stigmatized status.

The moral-religious identity of syphilis, alternately described as the Almighty's "registered stamp for the act of adultery," as a "salutary bridle" placed by Provi-dence on sexual immorality, and as the "wages of sin," was everywhere apparent within American society.[66] Broadcast through sermons, medical texts, novels, plays, and many other forms of popular culture, the era's hegemonic narrative cast syphilis as a "shameful disease" brought on by the "sin of unchastity."[67] While the rise of germ theory and bacteriology dislodged many other diseases from long-standing associations with immorality and sin, the growing conviction that sickness resulted from a violation of *nature's* laws (rather than God's) did not extend to syphilis. Simply put, this disease was "still under the banner of ostracism."[68]

The stigma surrounding syphilis had profound implications for the infected. For one, it prevented them from gaining admittance to hospitals, which rou-tinely shut their doors on syphilitic sufferers.[69] Privately practicing physicians sometimes also refused to treat VD, arguing that this would only remove "restraining influences to wrongdoing."[70] As one doctor opined, the "Supreme Intelligence" had created syphilis and gonorrhea to "develop the moral nature of man by demanding that he exercise will-power and restraint over his desires."[71] More sympathetic physicians condemned those "compassionless moral snobs" who could not "forget the moral deficiencies of his patient and think only of his sickness."[72] Nevertheless, most doctors had little interest in treating VD, and medical students received little to no training in the diagnosis and treatment of syphilis and gonorrhea.[73] Indeed, despite the emergence of venereology as a legitimate medical specialty during this period, the view that VD ought to be approached "from a purely scientific standpoint" was slow to gain ground.[74] As one aspiring, first-generation venereologist learned, it was "almost as disgraceful to treat syphilis as to contract it."[75]

With their access to public and private medical care severely restricted, those infected with syphilis had few opportunities for professional treatment. Even when available, most had little interest in consulting with venereologists. In part, this reluctance owed to the particular kinds of remedies most commonly employed in the treatment of syphilis: mercury and the iodides of potassium (often referred to as "potash"). Widely regarded as an "evil," as a therapeutic strategy akin to "jumping from a high window in order to escape a burning building," the general public so "hated and detested" mercury that many syphilitic patients either terminated courses of mercurial therapy shortly after their commencement or simply refused their administration altogether.[76] The cause of patients' opposition to this "most dangerous weapon" is not hard to fathom: even when given in smaller doses, the side effects of mercury commonly included gangrene, bone lesions, paralysis, and alopecia.[77] For their part, the iodides often led to headaches, sinus troubles, frequent head colds, cutaneous eruptions resembling acne, and a condition dubbed "iodism," by which practitioners referred to the "general nervous irritation, with depression (sometimes very extreme), caused occasionally in individuals by the use of iodide."[78]

Acknowledging their frequently "deplorable results" in the field of antivenereal care, VD specialists castigated the rank-and-file physician's unthinking, "futile and inadequate" manner of handling syphilis, arguing that "better education" of the general practitioner was something "imperatively demanded."[79] "The general ignorance of the medical profession regarding syphilis is deplorable," one VD specialist thundered, "and a reproach that we should feel."[80] Echoing these views, nonspecialists admitted that "the whole treatment of syphilis is unsatisfactory," confessing to "a great many mistakes . . . in the diagnosis and treatment of syphilis."[81] As one irate venereologist quipped, "If the medical profession knew more of [syphilis's] true pathological conditions," then "fewer . . . would have to send their patients to Hot Springs Arkansas to cover up their damnable blunders."[82]

Admissions such as these likely rang true for Archie Cowles. In spring 1907, before he left for Hot Springs, Cowles sought to alleviate the "terrible pain" he lived with every day by consulting a physician. His chief concern at this time was a sore throat, which he first complained of in a letter of October 1, 1905. Before his first trip to Hot Springs, Cowles's throat was already swollen with sores that made swallowing well-nigh impossible.[83] "If it gets much worse," he wrote to a friend on April 29, 1906, "I shall have to quit work . . . for it . . . hurts to drink . . . [and] I can't eat tomatoes or anything sour." After learning that these symptoms were the result of a venereal infection, Cowles's doctor dosed him with potassium iodide. While providing temporary relief, this doctor's visit left Cowles with "terrible dyspepsia, confusion of thought, unstrung nerves, and vital drains." In the end, it would only serve to "drive a few more nails in my coffin," he predicted in a letter dated June 23, 1906. Almost a year later, Cowles secured a second appointment. Its results were similarly unwelcome, as he reported in a letter of May 5, 1907. "The doctor burned out my throat," Cowles informed a friend, adding that "I should not let him if I had known. . . . I am taking four iodides—mercury, potash, iron, and arsenic. That ought to brace me up or kill me."

From here, Cowles's attitudes toward doctors only worsened. Not keen on reliving his first two experiences with the profession's drugs of choice in antisyphilitic therapy, while en route to Hot Springs, Cowles informed a fellow railway passenger, as he wrote in a July 14, 1907, letter, that "if I had my way, I would shoot 90% of the blankety-blank doctors at the Springs, so people could get the benefit of the baths." Only once during his time in Hot Springs did he consult a physician. When this doctor suggested the iodides of potassium, Cowles quickly turned on his heels, leaving the man's office in a state of disgusted shock. "It was useless to tell him I had taken it for years, and that it only suppressed the disease temporarily, and that I had taken it so long it made me crazy," Cowles wrote a friend on November 10, 1907. "If I had done as he said and had died or gone insane, he would have taken it as a matter of course and still sung the old parrot tune, 'iodide of potash,' but they know nothing better."

In addition to limiting their access to quality medical care, the stigma surrounding syphilis also had a more direct, personal impact. According to venereologists, the feelings of shame and guilt that accompanied the contraction of syphilis were so intense that the disease's victims were "afraid to be found taking medicine or making applications of any kind."[84] Indeed, numerous practitioners testified that syphilitics' "fear of detection" caused many cases of venereal disease to "remain untreated" in the United States each year, as shame and a desire to keep their illness a secret impelled sufferers to hide their infections from public view.[85]

Hoping to hide their diseases from family, friends, and neighbors, syphilitics frequently sought treatment far from home. Even within Hot Springs, some venereal health seekers were so afraid of having their illnesses publicly revealed that they "had their letters either addressed anonymously or mailed to some neighboring post office."[86] Nonresident doctors also recorded stories of health seekers using assumed names in Hot Springs, noting that these aliases were adopted so as to "conceal the fact of their being treated for syphilis."[87] For most, however, it was the respite from broader social discourses of blame and sin that made this remote Arkansas site appealing. As a Colorado doctor who visited the city observed, what made Hot Springs appealing was the fact that there was "no necessity of concealment" of a patient's condition there.[88] Echoing this, a colleague remarked that in Hot Springs, "the patient does not have to conceal his disease from everyone, and is not in constant dread that his ailment will be discouraged and he disgraced."[89] What Hot Springs offered first and foremost, then, was a means of "administering to minds diseased."[90]

Aware of the broader linkages between sex, disease, and sin, local doctors and entrepreneurs skillfully turned this discourse to their own ends, presenting Hot Springs as a spiritual haven that put health seekers in touch with forces of divine healing and forgiveness. Indeed, the connective tissue that linked syphilis to Hot Springs was highly spiritual in nature. Newspapermen declared the area "a boon to suffering humanity wrought by the hand of God," while government officials spoke of the "mysterious agents imparted to the water by the hand of the Deity."[91] Resort doctors attributed the springs' therapeutic prowess to "some specific work of Providence," with one even penning an epic poem entitled "The Vale of Healing Waters." This spiritual panegyric transported readers back to the moment at which "the God of generous wonders . . . breathed upon these sparkling waters," after which God decreed Hot Springs the place where "the sick of every station" should gather "for the healing of their illness."[92]

Local medical men ascribed supernatural healing powers not only to the springs but to the entire surrounding area. Speaking to the forests, rivers, and mountains that blanketed the region, they referred to Hot Springs as a place whose beautiful scenery called the mind "from nature up to nature's God"—as a city that counted its physical environment among those "natural advantages . . .

which the good Lord has seen fit here in his great wisdom to bestow upon us."[93] For the venereal health seeker, entering into this "perpetual Sabbath" was of decided benefit; once looking upon himself as "an outcast, with the mark of Cain on his brow," he would now "forget that he is afflicted with a loathsome disease."[94] Noting that "the scenery about the springs is wild and magnificent," one local observer explained that "many who go there are impressed with the belief that anything so wonderful must possess great curative powers."[95]

With the passage of time, this message traversed a wide variety of media— much of it created and disseminated by outsiders. Fraternal organizations and unions wrote of Hot Springs as a place whose "miraculous pools" had been graced by "the fingers of God" and where every day one witnessed cures "as wonderful as those of the days of the Saints and the sacred tales of the Scriptures, when the Angels appeared at Bethesda."[96] Perhaps inspired by local doctors, visiting physicians published religious odes about the city; one, a 1908 piece entitled "The Story of Hot Springs," explained how

> Here stood the work the Almighty God made,
>> Before man and his kind had come
> For blessed were the waters a kind God gave
>> In proof of His great love the sum. . . .
> And the site which still marks the 'fountain of youth'
>> As the blessing from God's good hand,
> Is the Hot Springs, thro' which has been fed
>> Good health to a suffering land.[97]

Another likened the resort to Lourdes, a famous French shrine with a reputation for miraculous cures.[98] And just as homegrown promotional efforts targeted the venereally infected, outside observers linked their biblically inspired assessments of the springs to VD. As one commentator put it, the city's waters "seem to act as favorably upon syphilitic cases as did the waters of Jordan in healing antique Lepers."[99] Others spoke of "syphilitic pilgrims" who "ben[t] the knee and worship[ped] devoutly" at the springs and who returned home to praise the "supernatural aid" they had received at these miraculous "wells of nature."[100]

Hot Springs' construction as a place where "salvation was to be found" had a tangible impact on the kinds of medicine practiced there.[101] Among other things, the city was home to a wide variety of "faith healers." One of the most well known of their number, a German-born mystic named Francis Schlatter, spent several months in Hot Springs during the late 1890s, and years after this, in a letter dated July 14, 1907, Archie Cowles recounted an encounter with another "Divine

Healer."[102] Describing him as a "tall and willowy" man with "pale blue eyes" and "fine blonde hair," this self-proclaimed miracle-worker performed his cures by seizing the wrists of his patients, "fix[ing] his eyes on heaven," and then "rub[bing] the back of their necks" until the relief of their affliction had been secured. Unsure of what to make of this resident holy man, the visitor wryly concluded that he supposed "they get some good out of it, for they have exchanged magnetism with a stronger character than themselves."

For those accustomed to thinking of their illnesses as the "wages of sin," the appeal of a place said to promise a "blessing" from "God's good hand" cannot be overlooked. Turn-of-the-century physicians regularly reported instances in which their syphilitic patients turned to "faith cure" as a means of recovering lost health, and religious rituals (notably fasting) played a prominent role in popular therapeutic behaviors surrounding this disease.[103] Though the medical profession was largely critical of these methods, it is clear that numerous individuals—authorities and patients alike—evidently preferred the "religious treatment" to "proper medical therapy."[104] Hot Springs was part of this broader quest for spiritual cures. In their attempts to promote medical travel to this central Arkansas resort, resident doctors, businessmen, and elected officials drew on the connections that had been established between syphilis and morality and religion, turning them to their own advantage by presenting the springs' antisyphilitic qualities as a gift bestowed on humanity by a merciful, compassionate God. For those taught to regard their ailments as a just punishment for immoral behavior, this message produced a strong response, as many of those who traveled to Hot Springs doubtless believed that being in the presence of the Almighty's handiwork would result in deliverance from both the physical and psychological symptoms of syphilis.

This is likely why so many visitors attached a spiritual significance to the springs' antisyphilitic energies. So enamored of its waters were these venereal health seekers, one late nineteenth-century observer reported, that on a daily basis syphilis-stricken patients could be seen at Hot Spring "bending the knee of worshiping devoutly this almost panacea."[105] Concurring with this assessment, those physicians favorably disposed toward the springs drew parallels between this modern-day therapeutic marvel and ancient biblical sites of healing.[106]

Physicians and medical observers regularly imparted a religious meaning to the experiences of the city's visiting syphilitics.[107] Their descriptions harken back to the sixteenth century, an era in which Europe's venereally afflicted sought the cure for syphilis through pilgrimages to sacred sites such as Dettelbach-on-the-

Main and the shrine of the Mother of God in the Thuringian Forest. Popularized by chroniclers such as Johannes Trithemius and Wilhelm Dersch, whose writings testified to the "miraculous cures" seen at such places, these and other holy sites quickly established a reputation among the venereally afflicted, inspiring them to pray to Minus, Anna, and the era's other patron saints of syphilis.[108]

Though some three-hundred years distant, the motives that underwrote the medical pilgrimages of America's turn-of-the-century syphilitics were not that different from those described by early modern writers like Trithemius and Dersch. While the ways in which Western societies thought about health and disease changed markedly between the mid-sixteenth and early twentieth centuries, people of both eras held to what one writer termed the "ancient conception" of syphilis—that it was God's "retribution for sins." Given the popular belief that it constituted "a stern curse of God against evil," for many of its sufferers the cure of syphilis necessitated a program of religiously oriented therapeutics, remedies that reflected its identity as a disease of the ungodly.[109]

To be sure, Hot Springs' "syphilitic pilgrims" did not always obtain the desired result. Nonresident observers frequently noted cases in which venereal health seekers were "made much worse" on account of their trips to Hot Springs.[110] Bathing in waters "hot enough to scald the devil" could be dangerous.[111] As numerous commentators observed, the hydrotherapeutic process essentially "shocked the whole nervous system from head to foot," increasing a patient's respiratory and heart rates while also taxing their internal organs.[112] Hoping to prevent any untoward results, the federal government advised that patients bathe only every other day "until they become acclimated."[113] Regardless, those who partook of the baths without supervision sometimes pressed their treatment to the "danger point," leading to "depressing and debilitating" effects such as exhaustion and fainting.[114] It was in part because of this that the resort fell into "rather bad repute" among certain medical professionals.[115]

From a present-day standpoint, the form of water cure practiced at Hot Springs might seem cruel and inhumane. Likened to "the lashing of the tides upon the sea-shore," its waters had the capacity to inflict bodily harm.[116] As historians of modern spas have demonstrated, however, this was widely accepted as just part of the treatment, with a "turn toward pain" characterizing nineteenth-century hydrotherapeutic cures.[117] During this period, spas all across Europe underwent a drastic transformation, as a new class of upwardly mobile urban professionals remade the continent's hydrotherapeutic resorts in their own image. Once associated with decadent, aristocratic excess, they were now thought to be bourgeois institutions thoroughly consistent with emerging middle-class values of productivity, modesty, and respectability. Hoping to discipline themselves and attain new levels of bodily self-regulation, spa goers resorted to a number of rather severe hydrotherapeutic procedures—from mud baths that produced intense burning sensations to steam baths capable of producing extreme "oppression and debility."[118]

While not vacationers by any stretch, the venereal health seekers of Hot Springs may have also sought a form of therapy bordering on punishment. Indeed, an unpleasant, chastising course of baths might have seemed essential to the alleviation of syphilis's psychological symptoms. It is perhaps for this reason that some described the springs in rather menacing terms—as something that, like a devilish cauldron, "boils and bubbles and hisses," that "laughs and dances in madcap revel."[119] If syphilis was the "wages of sin," the price to be paid for its cure might have been a course of physically painful therapy.

As all of this goes to show, syphilis's status as a stigmatized malady was not a deterrent to health seeking. Indeed, the actions of individuals such as Archie Cowles run contrary to the received wisdom on the relationship between medical stigma and patient behavior. In her influential *Illness as Metaphor* (1978) and *AIDS and Its Metaphors* (1989), cultural critic Susan Sontag contends that diseases with a shameful status actively discourage infected individuals from seeking out medical care. Internalizing society's judgmental attitudes toward them, Sontag argues, these sufferers adopt a mood of silent, fatalistic resignation that ultimately leads to death—even when life-saving treatments are available, a modus operandi that, according to Sontag, will persist until science succeeds in eradicating the "metaphors and myths" that underwrite religious and moralistic understandings of disease. Until then, these ideologies will *literally* "kill."[120]

Yet rather than encouraging the infected to remain untreated and to approach their illnesses with an attitude of silent, fatalistic resignation, the "wages of sin" discourse was in fact *productive*, generating curative behaviors that were consistent with syphilis's moral etiology.[121] Instead of yielding a "conspiracy of silence" that hindered the development of curative medicines, religious understandings of syphilis facilitated particular kinds of conversation about the disease, along with particular kinds of therapeutic responses to it.[122] Far from "killing" the sick, contemporary beliefs about syphilis's status as a shameful, disgraceful, loathsome disease instead shaped expectations as to what recovery and cure would look like.[123] Moreover, those beliefs were not universal, as some individuals were relatively unaffected by the "wages of sin" mentality.[124] In Hot Springs, venereal sufferers could not only obtain genuine relief from syphilis but also develop new, alternative etiological understandings of the disease.

To Live and Die in Peace

Like his fellow syphilitics, Cowles came to Hot Spring believing that the "prolonged use of the baths" would cure him.[125] Yet even if these hydrotherapeutic practices left him feeling "stronger," with the passage of time Cowles gradually acknowledged the difference between the rhetoric surrounding Hot Springs' "fountains of healing waters" and the reality so many syphilitics confronted within this community of the venereally afflicted. In a letter dated October 1, 1907, only a few months into his second stay, Cowles observed that while hundreds of his fellow venereal sufferers were "cured of . . . syphilis sufficiently to leave their crutches when they go home," many experienced only temporary relief, as "sooner or later back they come worse than ever, till finally a poison, rotten mass of flesh is dumped in a hole out in the old cemetery."

Sadly, such was the trajectory of Archie Cowles's second trip to Hot Springs. His condition steadily worsening, on August 24, 1907, Cowles wrote home to announce that he was "not so well," as "my eyes are becoming affected and there is still a chance of losing my nose or the roof of my mouth." While on this occasion he spared his readers the "unpleasant details," Cowles's subsequent letters proved more revealing. Describing the "uncanny things" syphilis had done to his body, in another letter dated November 10 Cowles explained how this disease "took the partition out of my nose, chewed my throat all to pieces, attacked the roof bone of my mouth and burrowed out along my right cheekbone," an unwelcome development leading him to equate the state of his bodily health to "rats gnawing a corpse." "Beginning with a small, deep hole no larger than [a] pin," his sores "quickly enlarge[d] into ragged edged fissures, running about one-half [of a] cupful of matter in a day." Describing himself as a "disfigured mental and physical wreck," it was at this point Cowles began to think that he would never leave Hot Springs. Continuing to experience numerous "bad spells," one year later a resigned Cowles wrote that he believed he would die in Hot Springs, writing on August 22, 1908, that it would be "my grave, living and dead."[126] Faced with what in his October 1 letter he called an "incurable disease," he was slowly being "eaten alive" by syphilis, a process the city's waters were powerless to stop.

Archie Cowles was not alone among those for whom Hot Springs' waters failed to provide the desired effect. According to the city's official records, some 136 individuals died of syphilis there between 1896 and 1917. Reflecting its status as a haven for Americans with syphilis, more than half of those who died from venereal disease were "visitors" to Hot Springs, and like Cowles, the overwhelming majority of these were white, middle-aged males.[127]

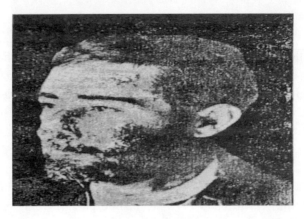

Though the historical record affords no visual documentation of Archie Cowles's time in Hot Springs, the man's own description of his physical symptoms closely matches those seen in this image, which comes from an advertisement for a popular turn-of-the-century antivenereal patent medicine. Courtesy of the Garland County Historical Society.

TABLE 1.1

Nonresident Deaths in Hot Springs Due to Syphilis, by Race, Sex, and Marital Status, 1896–1917

Race		Sex		Marital status	
White	56	Male	68	Married	19
Black	17	Female	5	Single	42
Total	73	Total	73	Total	61

As both the testimonies of eyewitnesses and its own vital statistics make clear, a significant proportion of Hot Springs' venereal health seekers ultimately succumbed to syphilis. Even if they did not recover, however, they did not give up. Instead of manifesting feelings of shame and guilt, instead of brooding over their diseases in withdrawn isolation, many of the city's syphilitics actively pursued each other's company, forging bonds of friendship that lifted their collective spirits and renewed their desire for life. While a belief that syphilis constituted the "wages of sin" may have both pushed and pulled them to Hot Springs, that ideology had little influence on the day-to-day lives of the resort's VD patients.[128]

Such was certainly the case for Archie Cowles. Though he regretted leaving Cleveland, Cowles quickly found both friends and time for leisurely diversions within Hot Springs. "I have got a little acquainted with a few people," he observed in a letter penned on July 31, 1907, a few weeks into his stay, adding that the buttons he brought with him from Cleveland were "great friend-finders." Whether taking baths or meals, Cowles was constantly in the company of other men, and so attached did he become to other visitors (whom he referred to as "our family" in a letter from February 4, 1906) that whenever a companion departed the resort, he eagerly hoped, as he wrote on July 14, 1907, to find a "congenial partner" among the next crop of medical tourists.

With these friends, Cowles engaged in all manner of diversions, as he described in a September 29, 1907, letter. On a regular basis, the members of his "happy family" trekked into town to see "religionists" and the various speakers who came to Hot Springs on the lecture circuit—including Kate Richards O'Hare, whose socialist views Cowles wholeheartedly sympathized with. During meals and in between treatments, Cowles frequently held forth on the subject of socialism; at one point, he had a friend ship him a collection of campaign materials in support of IWW founder Bill Haywood's anticipated presidential run. "The poor mortals that come here are hungry for reading matter and grab at a paper like a drowning man at straws," he wrote on July 31, 1907, adding that Hot Springs was "a grand place for propaganda work."

In addition to politics, health and medicine were frequent topics of conversation. Whenever a new group of neighbors took up residence in his hotel, Cowles, as he wrote on August 24, 1907, "got acquainted" with them by sharing stories about personal illness experiences. Jones "has a case of 'gon' of six years standing!" Cowles informed a friend about a Welshman that moved in next to him. "Mike has eczema, and Johnson has dropsy." Cowles described these and other acquaintances as "good friend[s]" with whom he was "quite chummy." During time spent together in bathhouses, he revealed in a January 12, 1908, letter, they had "fun . . . talking about the various medicines" different men and women sought out in Hot Springs—including remedies for syphilis. "Occasionally, some poor Reuben will begin to sing the praises of Dr. King's Golden Medical Discovery," Cowles wrote, remembering one particular conversation. "Then there is a derisive laugh from all, for everybody outside of Mayback Corners knows that Dr. K's GMD has about as much effect on a case of Syph as a flint arrow on an ironclad gunboat." Cowles also noted that "the good old Harem oil has quite a reputation here as a cure for Gon."

Of course, illness itself often intruded on these moments, and as their conditions worsened, health seekers often transformed into caregivers. After the Welshman named Jones became sick from a doctor who "tried to tear his prostate with a sound," Cowles wrote home on August 26, 1907, to explain that "I have to attend him some." On another occasion, Cowles befriended "an old German" with a "nearly rotted off" leg. Explaining in a July 31, 1907, letter that the man was a "harmless kind of lunatic," Cowles found that he had to "keep things clean after him," particularly as he could not pass a saloon without indulging his desire for alcohol. Through caring for individuals such as these, Cowles gained an understanding of his own illness and of the kinds of difficulties he could expect it to give rise to.[129]

In some ways, it appears that Cowles imbibed many of the era's stigmatized attitudes toward syphilis. A few months after arriving in the city for the first time, Cowles informed a friend (in a December 11, 1905, letter) that "if you will step down to Hot Springs I will show you a real chamber of horrors, no wax figures but living flesh and blood, where you can see not only bodies which are a mass of festering disease and mutilated forms, but also monstrosities and abnormalities of perverted sexuality, the results of ignorance and false teaching of parent or child, compelled by present social ethics as taught by orthodoxy and reinforced by conservatism." In another letter from August 24, 1907, Cowles spoke of the city's VD patients as "freaks and monstrosities" whose bodies were "so rotten as to hardly hold together." Hot Springs was a place where one beheld the results of "crimes as he never dreamed the existence of." "If you wish to know to what extent the various unnatural sex crimes are practiced at present," he relayed, "just come to Hot Springs and take a course of study."

In equating syphilitic patients with "freaks and monstrosities" guilty of perpetrating "unnatural sex crimes," Cowles may seem to be replicating the views of official guidebooks on Hot Springs, which recommended that parents send their "wild boys" to this "school" so as to receive a "good moral lesson." Yet while these texts emphasized individual reform aimed at "the preventing [of] their sowing wild oats," Cowles was much less personal, and much less moralistic in his assessment of the country's VD problems.[130] Whenever speaking of the "chamber of horrors" that greeted visitors to Hot Springs, he attributed their "festering" and "mutilated forms" not to moral improprieties but instead, to broader social, cultural, and economic factors. Attacking what he called in his August 24 letter the "conspiracy of ignorance and false doctrines" that surrounded syphilis, Cowles wrote on January 4, 1908, that the "unnatural sex crimes" that led to syphilis and gonorrhea were an inevitable product of "economic disorder" and of the "cruel, brutal, free moral agency doctrine" that taught sufferers that their conditions were a product of individual failures.

In his analysis of the country's struggle with VD, Cowles consistently set himself against those who, as he put it in an October 1, 1907, letter, "think men and women are bad because they love sin." He even defended sex workers in criticizing the system that led to the spread of the disease. While connecting his own suffering to the "bitterness of the prostitute," Cowles believed that the "increasing" number of "fallen women" within the United States was itself the product of a "systematic effort put forth to ruin working girls." Aligning himself with those Progressive reformers whose writings about the kidnapping and subsequent selling of young women into prostitution fueled a "white slavery" panic, he concluded that the only way to "check the terrible disease I have" was to pass and enforce laws capable of dismantling America's "vice trust."[131] Until society had "taken from the dollar its power to doom women to lives of shame," Cowles argued, young women would be continually "sacrificed on the altar of poverty, ignorance, and false morals."

Within Hot Springs, Cowles encountered little stigmatized behavior from the city's residents. During the end of his time there, he purchased forty acres of land and quickly set about clearing this for agricultural use and permanent residency. After constructing a dwelling, Cowles reported in a July 23, 1908, letter that he was "well fixed for neighbors." One, a man named "Mr. George," was a "good soul," and another, a "Mr. Cathey," was "kind and accommodating." After letting him settle in to his new abode, these neighbors brought Cowles the paperwork he needed to receive mail and even promised to bring him chickens for his farm. The actions of individuals who looked on syphilitics as a "national menace" these were not.

Cowles's experience in Hot Springs aligns with the testimonies of the city's medical practitioners. As one local doctor exclaimed, most of the resort's syphilitics arrived in a state of great "mental anguish," believing that they were "ruined for life."[132] But after a few days, something "magical" occurred. The health seeker's anxiety was "dispelled" and their minds put "at rest." The reason for this was clear, for "upon his arrival he finds so many fellow sufferers, and a number whose condition is so much worse than his own, that he consoles himself with the thought that it could have been worse. His unfortunate associates give him their moral support, resulting from a bond of brotherhood and sympathy that exists between them all. He has come to a 'haven of rest' where his trouble is treated as an accident instead of disgrace."[133]

Breathing an air free of stigma, Cowles found himself able to combat what he called in a November 10, 1907, letter the "mental pain" that constituted one of syphilis's most trying symptoms. "The thing I need most is peace of mind," he wrote on July 23, 1908, "[as I] can't stand worry." While "chummy" friends (August 22, 1908) and "kind" neighbors (July 18, 1907) helped on that front, so too did taking a lunch and a pail of water up through the Ozarks and spending his time writing in the comfort of cool mountain breezes.

"In spite of my infirmities," he declared on August 24, 1907, "I am a lover of nature," confessing that "when I get out of the city, the old love and enthusiasm comes back to me." On one particular occasion, Christmas Day 1907, Cowles "lit out" in the early morning, noting in a January 4, 1908, letter that he "went about three miles out [to] the Rock Island Railroad and sat down at the foot of the hill that is covered with a dense growth of young pines. A wide noisy stream made music," he continued, noting how "the grasshoppers, ants, and blue bottle flies made merry around me." These experiences, he concluded, left him feeling "pleasant" despite his loneliness; as Cowles relayed, "I enjoyed myself and wrote page after page." Such activities helped Cowles learn how to "live and die in peace," as he noted on August 22, 1908—something he would not have likely achieved absent traveling to Hot Springs. "Life is sweet even to me, a disfigured mental and physical wreck," he wrote on November 10, 1907. "I certainly love this old earth better than all the imaginary worlds that been invented, and I hope to come back here again to spend eternity."

Conclusion

In turn-of-the-century America, syphilis was regarded as the "wages of sin," and in many different ways, this belief conditioned Hot Springs' emergence as an asylum for Americans with syphilis. Working to push people with VD away from local sources of medical care, it also pulled them to this central Arkansas re-sort—a place said to be "medicated by the wisdom and power of the Benevolent and Almighty God for the healing of His *wayward people*."[134] The stigma attached to VD also played a part in determining which kinds of syphilitics traveled to Hot Springs; on account of society's comparatively tolerant attitudes toward white men with syphilis, members of this demographic predominated among the city's venereal health seekers. Syphilis's construction as an immoral malady also influenced the therapeutic choices of the disease's victims, as many who journeyed to Hot Springs sought relief not only from bodily suffering but also from the feelings of shame and guilt that accompanied the contraction of a heavily stigmatized malady. Partially on account of this, the cure of syphilis was closely attached to recovery from the disease's mental and emotional symptoms—a fact that made the resort a popular destination despite the high number of individuals who, like Archie Cowles, ultimately died of syphilis.

Despite this, however, it is clear that this disease was more than simply the "wages of sin." Within Hot Springs, at least, visiting health seekers constructed a relatively destigmatized place of healing, one where sufferers had the option to live free of guilt and shame. Caring for each other and receiving kind treatment at the hands of the city's local inhabitants, visiting patients constructed alternative etiologies for syphilis, which stressed not sin but bad luck, not immoral behavior but adverse social and economic circumstances. When looking at the "venereal peril" from the standpoint of individuals such as Archie Cowles, it becomes clear that instead of creating a "conspiracy of silence," turn-of-the-century Americans responded to VD in a way that was informed by networks of communication built up by syphilitic patients.

As the next chapter shows, this network included physicians as well. Syphilis was often portrayed as a classic disease of the "other," but in Hot Springs, doctors crafted a somewhat different identity for it, one associated with the conditions of urban, civilized life. Presenting their city as the antidote to the ills of the modern age, local doctors incorporated the curative strategies adopted by visiting syphilitics like Archie Cowles into their handling of syphilis, designing a system of antivenereal therapeutics that pinned the disease's treatment not so much to modern medical science as to a series of older, *hygienic* measures. In their hands, syphilis became something richer and more complex than has hitherto been recognized.

CHAPTER TWO

"Administering to Minds Diseased"

Treating Syphilis in Turn-of-the-Century Hot Springs

On July 29, 1904, Michael J. Murphy left his home in Palatka, Florida, and set out for Hot Springs, Arkansas. A forty-two-year-old businessman with a wife and two children, Murphy decided to traverse the nine hundred miles separating home from health resort because of a number of long-standing afflictions—gout, rheumatism, and a diseased kidney among them. Immediately after arriving, Murphy sought treatment at a local bathhouse, contracting the services of a doctor who agreed to treat his myriad medical problems. At the outset, Murphy was optimistic. "I think I shall get well here," he wrote home on August 5, adding that "I am feeling very comfortable."[1] A few days later, Murphy informed his wife that he was beginning to "feel strong," like his "old true self" (30). While subsequent weeks brought a number of setbacks, on August 25, he wrote that he was feeling "stronger" and that he would likely return home in a few weeks' time (68).

Unfortunately for Michael Murphy and his family, that return trip never occurred. On the night of August 30, an employee of the doctor treating him found Murphy lying on the ground in a "desolate spot" behind his hotel, bleeding profusely from cuts to the throat (78). The following morning, Murphy was pronounced dead. An official inquiry conducted by the city coroner concluded that he had died "from razor wound in left side of neck, self-inflicted while temporarily insane" (83). Days later, Murphy's family learned that he had "committed suicide . . . by cutting his throat with a razor" (86).

In their attempts to make sense of his death, those who testified before the city coroner linked Murphy's suicide to one crucial fact: he had been diagnosed with syphilis. According to those responsible for his care, upon arriving in Hot Springs, Murphy "did not know what was the matter with him" (78). After examining a sore in his groin, doctors concluded that his various ailments were all symptoms of an underlying syphilitic infection, which they treated with mercury and the iodides of potassium. Though his sore healed and he was reportedly "getting along very good," the diagnosis left Murphy mentally shattered (78). According to one witness, Murphy believed that "he was going to die from sickness" and "worried about his children coming along and it breaking out on them" (80–81). Others observed that his diagnosis "seemed to wear greatly on his mind." Often appearing "hysterical and unnerved," with the passage of time Murphy was said to have become "exceptionally despondent," eventually becoming so mentally unbalanced that, in a state of "temporary insanity," he chose to end his life (80). In strictly physical terms, however, Murphy "did not seem to [be] very sick at all" (81).

This version of events aligns with Murphy's own account. On the night of his death, Murphy penned a suicide note attempting to explain his state of mind. "I cannot stand the strain, my brain is one fire," he cried. "I have tried to turn to God," Murphy continued, "but I am too feeble. My brain is wracked. My wife and I never quarreled. I loved my family. O'God I love them but my brain is snapping. A suicide grave. My eyes are closing with the fearful pain in them. I see no way to escape. Have had no sleep for almost a week. This agony is more than I can stand" (76). In this agony, Murphy saw no other option than to carry out what he regarded as "my most terrible crime." In his last communication with the world of the living, he prayed that God and his family would forgive him for "this awful work" (76).

In many ways, Michael J. Murphy's sorrowful stay in Hot Springs echoes that of Archie Cowles. Both men traveled to Hot Springs from distant locations in the first decade of the twentieth century, and both received treatment for syphilis (although only Cowles explicitly journeyed here for that reason). Neither man recovered. And, perhaps most interestingly, both Cowles and Murphy experienced syphilis as an ailment of both body and mind, one that brought with it agony, despair, sadness, and regret. Taken together, the firsthand accounts of Cowles and Murphy provide some sense of syphilis's meaning in turn-of-the-century Hot Springs. As one local practitioner expressed it, "no other disease has evoked such mental agony" as syphilis, which "in not a few instances has driven its victim to a suicide's grave."[2]

There is, however, one crucial difference in Murphy's story. Whereas Archie Cowles went out of his way *not* to be treated by resort doctors, Murphy deliberately sought them out. In his first letter home, Murphy told of how he "had a talk with the Dr.," who told him that he could "be cured" (10). Throughout his stay, Murphy regularly updated his wife on the course of therapy (which included both drugs and surgical operations) he was undergoing, peppering his remarks with comments on the effects of his doctor's care. His letters, then, open a window onto the city's physicians—onto their own understandings of syphilis, their methods of diagnosis, their curative strategies, and professional behaviors. Murphy's correspondence offers an opportunity to probe the medical management of syphilis in turn-of-the-century America, and to examine this disease from the perspective of clinical practice.

Historians have yet to explore this aspect of the era's "venereal peril" in much depth. Existing accounts focus largely on public health responses to VD and on the ideologies embedded in the era's venereal discourse. In part, this oversight owes to the assumption that therapeutic approaches to syphilis and gonorrhea were "secondary" to moral and behavioral ones.[3] But as the experiences of people like Michael Murphy show, doctors played an important part in the country's antivenereal efforts. How did they perceive VD? How did they react to it? And to what extent did their curative efforts reflect broader debates about the relationship between sex, sin, and science?

Michael Murphy's letters offer some insight into these questions. Prior to his untimely death, Murphy not only was treated with conventional antisyphilitic remedies such as mercury and potassium iodide but also embraced methods more in keeping with the resort's broader therapeutic culture. Among them were the city's far-famed waters. Shortly after arriving, Murphy wrote of how he was "taking baths under order of a Dr" (21). Throughout his stay in Hot Springs, he regularly reported on how this activity—especially when combined with steady imbibing of the springs themselves—left him feeling "first rate" (29). In addition to this, Murphy was advised to "take all the exercise one can," whether it be climbing atop the region's "steep hills" or simply walking through town (33). And throughout his time in Hot Springs, Murphy's doctors forbade the consumption of alcohol. "[I] do not drink any beer or liquors, nor do I want them," he informed his wife on August 8 (21). Just before taking his life, Murphy explained that he had "not tasted whiskey, beer, or anything in that line" since he had arrived (73).

The doctor who treated Michael Murphy was but one among dozens of local, licensed private practitioners who earned their livelihoods treating syphilitic health seekers. And the medical care he received was representative of that offered by Hot Springs' de facto venereal specialists. Referred to as "hygienic treatment," this brand of medicine simultaneously targeted syphilis's symptoms and the immoral behaviors resident healers saw as the disease's ultimate cause. While mercury, baths, and other medical remedies were administered to arrest syphilis's physical and mental manifestations, a series of drugless measures (including prohibitions against drinking, smoking, gambling, sex, and other vices) served to restore the patient's moral conscience. A complex curative system, the "hygienic treatment" of syphilis brought both bodily healing and the return to a more godly, virtuous, and upright lifestyle. Its existence illustrates the value of examining medical practices, for whereas most historians cast the era's response to VD as a battle of "sin vs. science," the clinical behaviors of the city's physicians suggest that this conceptual framework is somewhat of a false dichotomy, one that overlooks the important ways in which "moral" and "biomedical" views of disease overlapped and aligned with each other.[4] Within Hot Springs, at least, there was no strict divide between "sin" and "science."

Attending to therapeutic matters also allows for a more complex understanding of the relationship between medicine, racial identity, and professionalization. Hygienic therapy did not appear in a vacuum. Both a therapeutic and an *ideological* response to illness, it was as much about healing the sick as it was about buttressing the moral status of Hot Springs' overwhelmingly white clientele—and by extension, the professional status of white resort doctors. Receiving a venereal diagnosis threatened to cast health seekers like Michael J. Murphy into the ranks of African Americans, who in the decades after the Civil War came to be regarded as a "syphilis-soaked" race.[5] In turn, specializing in the treatment of this disease had the potential to tarnish doctors' reputations, as many in both the lay and medical communities saw venereology as a disreputable pursuit—something for the uneducated charlatan rather than the respectable physician. Hygienic therapy was a solution to these problems: resort doctors were able to use it to carve a color line through VD, thereby preserving white patients' racial hegemony and successfully asserting their own medical authority over syphilis.[6] In so doing, they crafted a style of medical practice whose impact was felt far beyond Hot Springs.

The Healers of Hot Springs

The existence of a medical corps in Hot Springs dates back to the immediate postbellum period, when dozens of physicians and surgeons previously employed by the Confederate and Union militaries settled there in an attempt to take advantage of its burgeoning trade in medical tourism.[7] Within a decade of the Civil War's end, the growing city was home to dozens of licensed medical men, many of whom had graduated from prestigious schools (including Bellevue Hospital Medical College, the New York College of Physicians and Surgeons, the University of Virginia, and Tulane University) and been formally admitted into the American Medical Association.[8] With the passage of time, some of these doctors became university academics, publishing articles in local and national medical journals and achieving various degrees of notoriety.

Among their number was James T. Jelks. Arriving in Hot Springs in 1877, Jelks was a member of the American Association of Obstetricians and Gynecologists. Over the course of the next twenty-five years, he established himself as one of the country's foremost venereologists, occupying a chair as professor of genito-urinary surgery and venereal diseases at Chicago's College of Physicians and Surgeons (1883–1890) before becoming a lecturer in gynecology and syphilology at Barnes Medical College in St. Louis—all while maintaining a practice in Hot Springs.[9]

Another of the city's most successful first-generation physicians was James M. Keller. In 1877, Keller left his position as chair of Surgery at the Kentucky School of Medicine and Louisville Medical College to become a practicing physician at Hot Springs, where he remained until his death in 1914. In the intervening thirty-seven years, Keller organized the Hot Springs Medical Society, a professional association of the city's licensed doctors, and established the *Hot Springs Medical Journal*—a periodical highlighting the work of local physicians. Described as "a man of considerable force," Keller also established a reputation outside of Hot Springs, serving on the American Public Health Association's Committee to Prevent Venereal Diseases and as the vice president of the American Medical Association's section on dermatology and syphilis.[10] The author of many publications, eminent surgeons across the United States referenced his studies even after his death.[11]

Keller's initiatives within Hot Springs helped many of the city's white doctors advance their careers, but they hindered those of its black doctors. Although the city was home to a number of African American physicians, they were prohibited from joining the Hot Springs Medical Society and from publishing papers in the *Hot Springs Medical Journal*. Northern visitors to the resort expressed surprise at finding a color line "so distinctly drawn" through Hot Springs' medical institutions, but the form of Jim Crow seen here was common throughout the postbellum South.[12]

In the face of segregation and overt racial hostility, black practitioners struggled mightily to establish viable practices. One of the most successful among them was Claude Melnotte Wade, a dental surgeon who graduated from Central Tennessee College in 1888 and thereafter moved to Hot Springs. After a decade of practice within the city, Wade presented a paper at a meeting of the Arkansas Colored Medical Association decrying how "the negro doctor, to succeed, must succeed in spite of enemies, in spite of his friends, and oftimes in spite of himself."[13] Whenever unable to perform a miracle of healing at the bedside, Wade recounted, stories of how "the negro doctor killed him" resounded throughout the city—despite the fact that white doctors had likely also failed to improve the patient's condition.[14]

Wade was also intimately acquainted with the prejudices of the resort's white healers and castigated those who shut black doctors out of the medical profession's "sacred conclaves."[15] As he saw it, such a policy deprived potential colleagues of an opportunity to learn about the treatment of black patients, as healers such as himself were "more in touch" with those maladies that were "the heirlooms of slavery and superstition."[16] Despite his inability to fraternize with white doctors, Wade persisted, and in 1900 became owner of the Saint Pythias Sanitarium—a bathhouse with twenty beds that existed "for the care of sick and indigent colored people who come to Hot Springs."[17] Overcoming at least some of the innumerable hardships confronting black doctors, Wade maintained a local practice through the 1920s, by which time he had become one of the chief proponents of the "Hot Springs treatment."[18]

Though he regarded himself as "the oldest established colored physician in the city," Wade was not Hot Springs' sole black doctor.[19] Others included R. L. Torrence, who operated the city's Crystal Bath Palace for black health seekers, and Harold Phipps, who authored a number of papers on the subject of venereal diseases. Together, these three doctors were part of a growing group of middle-class black professionals who prospered in a city marked by the institutionalized racism of the Jim Crow South.

If James Keller and Claude Wade occupied one end of the spectrum of healers active in turn-of-the-century Hot Springs, at the other lay a group of unlicensed, uncredentialed medical workers. These ranged from faith healers like Francis Schlatter to the makers of patent medicines such as Lopez, Lower's Hot Springs Blood Remedy, and Society Salve. These products were marketed as "purely vegetable" in origin, and directly played into public distaste for the medical profession's drugs of choice in the treatment of syphilis.[20] Advising health seekers to "beware of ointments . . . that contain mercury," patent medicines were quite popular among visiting syphilitics; after dosing himself with a nostrum called Salvar, for example, Archie Cowles proclaimed this "an ideal remedy," noting how under its influence, "my blood circulated free and warm, and I slept fine."[21] According to one early twentieth-century visitor, every year, "millions of dollars" were spent on patent medicines within Hot Springs, "the only claim for which is that they cure venereal diseases."[22] As late as 1919, by which time the federal government had begun a campaign to eradicate all forms of medical charlatanry within the city, public health officials testified that instead of going to licensed physicians, "a large percentage" of health seekers were "purchasing remedies in drug stores and writing to advertising specialists for treatment."[23]

It was not only the presence of patent medicine vendors that prompted some to label Hot Springs a city "full of quacks and charlatans."[24] Rivalries among educated practitioners also produced similar charges. Perhaps the most notable professional dispute of the late nineteenth century centered around a doctor named Almon Brooks.[25] After moving to Hot Springs in 1867, Brooks set up a private practice and quickly built up a large clientele among the resort's syphilitic patients. So successful was he that Brooks eventually forged a business partnership with several other doctors from his home state of Virginia.[26] Not long after this, however, he ran afoul of another of the city's "pioneer doctors," a man named George Lawrence. A graduate of the University of Pennsylvania who was twice elected as a delegate to the American Medical Association, Lawrence and several colleagues accused Brooks of being a "professional fraud," someone who—despite the University of Virginia diploma that hung from the wall of his office—had only "informally graduated in the profession."[27] On numerous occasions during the early 1870s, Brooks was accused of "conduct unbecoming a physician."[28] According to one colleague, he exhibited a certain "contemptible aggressiveness," acting in a "boastful" manner toward patients and attempting to steal them from other resort doctors.[29] Echoing this, another resident MD felt him "guilty of eschewing all courtesy and honor belonging to our professional code," and a third accused him of parading a "racy letter" before his patients.[30] In 1877, the state medical association formally heard the charges against him, and after much discussion, Brooks was officially censured. Not long after this, he sold his business and moved to Chicago, where he became known as the "Hot Springs Specialist."[31]

The debate over whether Almon Brooks was a counterfeit MD speaks to the porous, fluid, fuzzy distinctions between charlatanry and professionalism in turn-of-the-century Hot Springs. More of a tool wielded to denigrate one's rivals than an accurate categorization of the methods utilized by different kinds of medical workers, the term "quackery" functioned as a boundary-making device that, far from describing reality, simply constructed *ideals* about what constituted ethical, professional conduct.

The promotional strategies of resort doctors give the lie to the idea that only uneducated or unlicensed healers violated these ideals. After the Civil War, the leaders of the American Medical Association increasingly saw commercial advertising as anathema to respectable practice, and as part of an effort to elevate themselves above the numerous "spermatorrhea quacks and venereal charlatans" who solicited business through newspapers and other forms of print media, elite doctors all across the country gradually forswore this kind of promotional activity.[32] Yet in Hot Springs, advertising remained a popular practice. Often, advertisements drew attention to a doctor's skills in the treatment of VD, promising that "the errors of youth" would be "corrected" or boasting of "the absolute cure of syphilis in all of its stages."[33] While notices such as these might seem a hallmark of the unlicensed, it bears noting that professional MDs also turned to newspapers to draw patients to their offices. Indeed, even such an esteemed physician as James Keller took advantage of this commercial opportunity, at one point informing prospective patients that "it is useless for syphilitics to come here unless they come determined to stay at least ten weeks."[34]

Behaviors such as these, as well as doctors' employment of "drummers," attracted the ire of the profession's elite.[35] In the national medical press, authorities regularly accused local healers of "unethical conduct," arguing that drumming and newspaper advertising had "thoroughly commercialized" them.[36] These charges threatened to undercut resort doctors' claims of professional status—while also depriving them of prospective patients. Indeed, so damaging was the insinuation that the city consisted solely of "pseudo-practitioners and unscrupulous vendors of medicine" that around the turn of the century, local medical leaders mounted a campaign to improve resort doctors' standing in the eyes of the broader American medical community.[37]

This campaign was multipronged and involved a crackdown on drumming and newspaper advertising. At its center lay a federal committee created "for the control of the practice of medicine in Hot Springs." Consisting of a board of experts who examined resort doctors "as to their qualifications to prescribe the use of the hot waters," the committee introduced a system of medical governance into the city.[38] Those judged competent would be formally admitted to the Hot Springs Medical Society and have their names formally published in the *Hot Springs Medical Journal*—which also pledged itself to "weeding and stamping out the irregular and unprofessional practices" common to the region, practices that threatened to "mar the reputation of this, the greatest sanitarium on the continent."[39] Through such measures, local medical professionals sought to "elevate the standard of practice in Hot Springs," to "remove the odor of commercialism which for so long has stigmatized the medical profession of the 'City of Vapors.'"[40]

The extent to which these reforms advanced resort doctors' legitimization project is questionable. While the ethics crusade launched by local medical leaders produced some notable results, it failed to uproot nonresident doctors' negative assessments of Hot Springs. The very fact that Hot Springs was populated by thousands of sexually diseased individuals was enough to convince many Americans that the city was desperately in need of "cleansing and purifying."[41] Indeed, while the springs themselves were said to flow directly from the hand of God, the city built around them was often understood by way of another, countervailing biblical image: that of a "modern Sodom."[42] Inhabited by patent medicine dealers and unscrupulous healers, Hot Springs was also said to be the home of "grafters" and "lewd women" whose gambling houses and brothels "infested" the city. For these "moral vampires," Hot Springs was a "paradise"; for everyone else, it was a "plague spot."[43] Attitudes such as these provided the context within which local healers crafted their unique therapeutic response to syphilis.

The Hygienic Treatment of Syphilis

Regardless of their level of education or professionalism, there was one thing that united Hot Springs' myriad healers: the treatment of syphilis. Seeing that an "unduly large proportion of persons infected with syphilis come to Hot Springs for treatment," local medical men believed that "no other medical school in America" afforded as much material for "clinical instruction" on venereal disorders as did this central Arkansas health resort.[44] Because it presented "a great deal of syphilis," Hot Springs offered "a better opportunity [for] observing the horrors of [this] disease" than any other place in the United States, and as there was "no other city" in which to study it "in so many interesting and varied phases," resident physicians considered themselves experts in the treatment and cure of this venereal malady.[45] Boasting of their therapeutic skills, the healers of Hot Springs promised to restore the syphilis-stricken to health within a "very short time." "Can the physician in the ordinary lines and places of practice," one local doctor taunted, "make good any such promises as these?"[46]

In some ways, the brand of syphilitic therapy practiced in turn-of-the-century Hot Springs was no different than that offered by the broader American medical community. Like physicians elsewhere, the city's resident healers made great use of the profession's drugs of choice in the treatment of syphilis: mercury and the iodides of potassium.[47] According to one report, roughly ten thousand pounds of mercury annually found its way into the bodies of the city's syphilitic population.[48] It did so largely through a technique known as "inunction," by which a rubber mitt was used to spread mercurial ointment across a patient's back. One resident practitioner described the process in detail: "The patient usually takes his bath some time after breakfast, then repairs to the 'rubbing parlor,' where the inunction is given. The patient sits astride a chair facing the back, folds his arms on it and places his chin on his arms, the rubbing continuing for twenty to twenty-five minutes. He then puts on a thin undershirt, which is used as a 'mercury shirt,' for one week without change, the inunction usually being given daily."[49] This procedure, declared a prominent venereologist after a visit to the city, represented "the prevailing method at the Springs."[50]

While physicians prescribed this treatment, the actual curative work of inunction was performed by local bathhouse attendants—the overwhelming majority of whom were black.[51] A dirty, disagreeable form of labor that was generally "shun[ned]" by the city's white inhabitants, the position of "mercury rubber" nevertheless required a great deal of knowledge and skill.[52] In order to enter this line of work, prospective attendants needed to first complete a training course conducted at the free bathhouse run by the government. Even after obtaining employment at a private bathing facility, the medical director of the Hot Springs Reservation had the power to remove anyone who failed to adequately perform their duties.[53] On account of their many years of service, many bathhouse attendants became medical experts in their own right—not only with regard to the general principles of personal hygiene but also in connection with syphilis.[54]

One particular example of this can be seen in the case of a bathhouse worker named Henry Davenport, who attended to one Elijah Price. Price, a Minnesota lumberman, traveled to Hot Springs in 1899 and 1900 and the next year tragically died in a fire. Shortly thereafter, his mother tried to collect on a life insurance policy Price had purchased from the Standard Life and Accident Insurance Company. When they denied her request, her family took the company to court, and during a hearing, representatives of Standard Life and Accident informed a Minnesota Supreme Court judge that Price had lied to them when he took out his policy. Though he had declared himself of sound mind and body, officials believed that Price's trips to Hot Springs indicated a preexisting illness of a chronic nature.

Their evidence for this came from Davenport's testimony, whose deposition in the case was taken in Hot Springs. A twenty-six-year-old native of Hot Springs who had worked in various bathhouses for more than a decade, Davenport recalled giving Price "over twenty-one baths" during his time at the resort.[55] Asked whether he thought his patient was suffering from syphilis, Davenport responded in the affirmative, explaining that the man's paralyzed arm and the mercury observed on his body both pointed in this direction. During cross-examination, attorneys for the Price family questioned this conclusion and challenged Davenport's claims to be able to distinguish the symptoms of syphilis from those of other diseases. In response, Davenport informed the court that while he lacked a formal medical education, he had read several medical books and had learned about syphilis from "the medical journals around here in Hot Springs."[56] Moreover, as someone who had "handled barrels" of mercury, Davenport felt confident in his ability to accurately identify patients who had been treated with this substance.[57] "For one using it around like I was and as frequently as I was," he testified, "I could rub my hand over anyone's back in the dark and tell whether he had been rubbing or not."[58]

Perhaps sensing that their case was in jeopardy, at this point in the proceedings, Price's legal team decided to draw attention to Davenport's race. The members of the Minnesota court would not have the opportunity to interview him personally, the plaintiff's attorney explained, and though the question filled him with "regret," he nevertheless felt compelled to ask Davenport to "state whether you are a colored man." "I am a negro, born this way," he responded, adding that he had known only two white bathing attendants during his career in Hot Springs.[59] Unfortunately for the Prices' lawyers, this attempt at race baiting proved unsuccessful, as local physicians similarly testified that "syphilis is a very common cause of paralysis."[60]

Despite the fact that the resort's mercury rubbers were skilled, knowledgeable medical practitioners, the treatment they received from white health seekers was sadly often similar to that which Davenport received from the Prices' legal experts. Like the black doctors who faced accusations of having "killed" patients who died under their care, bathers who fell prostrate or experienced an "excessive reaction" often blamed their misfortunes on "the negligence of [the] bath attendant."[61] Even those who emerged unscathed from the bathhouse sometimes complained about their "strong-armed" African American attendants, whose "profuse perspiration" was evidently a most "distressing" feature of the experience.[62] Others accused their attendants of cheating them out of money or time.[63]

In reality, whatever harm the bathhouse experience yielded was much more likely to affect mercury rubbers than their patients. Local white doctors claimed that inunction was an entirely safe procedure, attesting that in decades of practice, they had never seen any signs of "mercurial poisoning" among attendants.[64] Nonresident venereologists concurred that they had "never seen any ill results to rubbers," though some cautioned that those who feared mercurialization might don rubber gloves so as to protect their hands.[65] The fact that this practice was widely adopted in Hot Springs suggests that mercury rubbing was a potentially hazardous occupation; indeed, a number of contemporary studies documented how medical workers employed in hospitals "became salivated" (that is, experienced increased salivation in the mouth) after patients were given the inunction treatment.[66] Within Hot Springs, a 1903 report issued by the reservation super-intendent conceded that mercury rubbing was a "hazardous business and de-structive of health."[67] The threat of mercurial poisoning was just another in a long line of slights and injustices African American bathhouse attendants were subjected to. And yet, despite these difficulties, some managed to parlay the in-come from this unpleasant occupation into great personal and professional success.[68]

Typically, bathhouse attendants kept up this course of inunction for two months, over which time the average syphilitic patient received thirty "rubs." With each inunction containing between an eighth and a sixth of an ounce of mercury, it was not uncommon for patients to leave Hot Springs having had ten or more ounces of the "blue ointment" rubbed into them.[69] As physicians inside and outside the city recognized, the Hot Springs method was a most heroic kind of therapy, one that relied on "large doses" of mercury.[70] Yet while such a form of antisyphilitic treatment elsewhere only worsened a patient's condition, at Hot Springs the "large doses" approach apparently worked wonders: "Under this form of administration," remarked a visiting naval surgeon, "I have seen lesions that have resisted every form of medication, heal and disappear as if by magic."[71]

The key to Hot Springs' "magic" in the treatment of syphilis was its boiling waters. Conducted via iron pipes into local bathhouses, the region's sizzling streams and steamy pools were employed to facilitate the elimination of chemi-cal toxins, which enabled syphilitic patients to withstand much higher levels of mercury than would be otherwise possible.[72] Making extensive use of this hybrid therapy, resident physicians marveled at how their patients' symptoms "dis-appeared promptly under the influence of the baths and specific medication in a very short time."[73] A bath a day, they contended, kept "the cumulative and bad effects of the mercury" away.[74]

Interestingly, however, despite the encouraging results it reportedly yielded, the local response to syphilis consisted of much more than a combination of chemical and hydro therapies. Indeed, as resort doctors saw it, "far too many phy-sicians confine[d] themselves to treating the disease with mercury and the io-dides."[75] The physician's "first line" of attack against syphilis, they reasoned, had to be of a drugless nature—something capable of keeping the patient "in a con-dition able to resist [its] ravages."[76] That something, which did "not receive the at-tention" it should have "at the hand of the general practitioner or the specialist in our towns and cities," was the "hygienic treatment of syphilis."[77]

"Hygiene" was the cornerstone of local responses to syphilis. According to resident doctors, the average venereal health seeker was "not leading a life

conforming to the laws of hygiene."[78] Therefore, it was "of the utmost importance . . . to look after the hygiene of the patient."[79] Doing this meant ensuring that patients ate "plain" foods, avoided "stimulants of all kinds," indulged
in "exercise in the open air," and took at least "eight hours' sleep" each night.[80]
It also meant prohibiting sexual activity; the syphilitic patient was "not [to] be
allowed to indulge his sexual appetite under any circumstances."[81] Such a regimen was designed to improve the patient's "mental condition" and bring about a
certain "personal reformation."[82] "Morbid habits must be broken up by firm but
gentle moral treatment," one local medical man exclaimed.[83] Patients needed to
be "treated psychologically," his colleagues concurred: syphilis could only be
cured through "hygiene and the great moral principle of right."[84]

This emphasis on moral treatment reflected syphilis's status as the "wages of
sin," along with local healers' own religious convictions. Speaking to these, in
1893, James Jelks presented a paper at the American Medical Association entitled
"The Antiquity of Syphilis, and Moses as a Health Officer." An analysis of the
Baal Peor plague of Old Testament times, the paper contended that the disease
that afflicted the ancient Israelites as they journeyed through the wilderness was
"frankly and purely syphilis" and had been visited on them after they incurred
the "wrath of Jehovah" by "falling into fornication with the daughters of Moab."[85]
In his talk, Jelks praised Moses's handling of the epidemic, which included having twenty-four thousand men who had slept with Moabite women killed and
promulgating a series of laws that forbade incest, bestiality, prostitution, homosexuality, and other forms of "improper" sexual relations among the Israelites.[86]
These measures were, according to Jelks, Moses's "rules of hygiene"; it was Moses's "enforcement of scrupulous cleanliness" among the Israelites, he concluded,
that led to the eventual "extinction" of the plague of Baal Peor.[87]

As they did for Moses, the healers of Hot Springs linked their success in the
treatment of syphilis to their preference for hygienic measures. The reason VD
patients "improve so much more rapidly than elsewhere," they concluded, owed
to their greater "control over such cases," which allowed them to remove the "influence of bad associations"—including "spirits, narcotics, and tobacco in every
form."[88] Unlike elsewhere, in Hot Springs the syphilitic sufferer obeyed the physician "absolutely": "If we tell him to stop using tobacco he will do it. If he has
been accustomed to alcoholic drinks he will not touch them. If he has been dis-
sipating by keeping later hours, he will retire at any time we tell him. If the plea-
sures of the table are a temptation to him, on the order of his physician he will
lead an abstemious life. In other words, we can have him under perfect control
and we may do with him whatsoever we like."[89] These "hygienic" habits were dif-

ficult to maintain outside of Hot Springs, where "the morbid eagerness for excitement and gain" were "too strong to be warded off" by the venereally afflicted.[90]

The emphasis local doctors placed on hygiene set them apart from nonresident medical men. In their advice to the broader profession, venereal specialists often recommended that syphilitic patients modify their diets, abstain from alcohol, and obtain more rest than would otherwise be the case. However, "moderate" levels of indulgence were permitted.[91] To insist otherwise, venereologists counseled, would only hinder treatment; as one writer explained, "the hygienic routine must not . . . be made so irksome that the patient will rebel and refuse to continue."[92]

In Hot Springs, however, doctors' "strict regimen" and "rigid hygienic rules" apparently produced "magic" results.[93] The syphilitic "whose mode of life is unhygienic" and could not be "controlled" at home, medical observers noted, was often markedly benefited by a sojourn at the springs, as there those "addicted to excesses" typically set aside any and all vices.[94] In their own reports, venereologists remarked that while in Hot Springs, the syphilitic patient "sedulously refrains from alcoholics, from tobacco, from the card table with its late hours, and from sexual indulgence." This "personal reformation" played a "very important part" in the sometimes surprising cures seen there.[95] According to one Chicago doctor, while at Hot Springs the syphilitic was "relieved of the temptation to drink, to smoke, to become indiscreet in diet or habits," and on account of this "he progresses more satisfactorily."[96]

Syphilis, Moral Treatment, and Race

Although resident and nonresident physicians similarly celebrated hygienic therapy's effects, its results were often quite disappointing. In their own reports, resort doctors conceded that a "goodly per cent" of Hot Springs' venereal health seekers left their offices only to "continue lives of dissipation and excess," returning year after year to "make amends for their injudicious living."[97] Indeed, local healers' experiences daily reminded them that "all mankind is weak and little to be trusted."[98] Yet despite the frequent setbacks they met with, doctors pursued this regimen without hesitation; as one put it, the cure of syphilis required them to exert a "psychic influence," to "be to all men a moral guide."[99]

The emphasis resort healers placed on being "moral guides" was consistent with broader trends in southern medicine. During the nineteenth century, medical graduates all across the region learned that establishing a successful practice required them to mix the voice of the scientist with that of the moralist, as many patients believed that being a good doctor first and foremost meant being a *good man.* Responding to the preferences of the communities in which they served, southern MDs developed a style of clinical practice that delicately merged science with morality and that foregrounded their roles as "mentors of sorts."[100] The success of this professionalization strategy, which persisted into the postwar period, doubtless convinced Hot Springs' resident physicians that in order to acquire medical authority, they would have to present themselves as "moral practitioners."[101]

Hot Springs' reputation as a "maelstrom of vice" gave resort doctors an additional reason for brandishing their moral credentials.[102] Officials in charge of the Hot Springs Reservation regularly received complaints that the city was more of a gambling resort than a health resort, and hoped that through their reforms "the moral tone of the place can be bettered."[103] But with gambling establishments, brothels, and other "questionable houses" beyond the bounds of government property, there was little they could do to alter the "dark picture" many had of the city.[104] Thus, it fell largely to doctors to counter the prevailing belief that it was "dangerous to come here."[105] Accentuating the resort's positive moral qualities, hygienic therapy was the right tool for the job.

Syphilis's status as a disease of sexual immorality gave doctors yet another reason for stressing their roles as "moral guides." Though often unsuccessful in convincing their patients to abstain from drinking, smoking, gambling, or sexual intercourse, doctors' insistence on "personal reformation" served to demonstrate the strength of their own moral convictions to the broader medical community. In proclaiming syphilitics' capacity to correct certain "morbid habits," they also rebutted the popular conception that Hot Springs was a place of "lascivious living"—the place where "the aged sinner and the youthful debauchee meet."[106]

Yet there were limits to doctors' advocacy of moral regeneration. A project of racial boundary making as much as it was a curative regimen, hygienic therapy was designed explicitly for white health seekers, whose syphilitic infections threatened association with the myriad "others" typically blamed for the country's VD problems.[107] By directing attention toward the disease's psychological attributes, hygienic treatment offered white patients a means of maintaining their social and cultural hegemony, preserving their sense of superiority over the group most often associated with syphilis in the US South: African Americans.

As the nineteenth century neared its end, southern medical men increasingly associated venereal disease with blacks, whom many referred to as a "syphilis-soaked race."[108] Prior to the Civil War, these physicians argued, slavery's "forced system of hygiene" had made syphilis "an unknown disease among the Negroes."[109] But with emancipation, former slaves flocked to cities and towns, and syphilis became "one of the most common diseases" among them.[110] The reason for this was clear: without an owner to govern their behavior, black men and women gave free rein to their sexual appetites, sowing and reaping diseases wherever they went.[111]

Interestingly, however, it was thought that they contracted a quite different form of venereal disease than did white men and women.[112] Among the myriad symptomological differences doctors documented between the two groups, the most frequently commented on concerned those late-stage complications of syphilis characterized by deterioration of the nervous system, brain damage, and mental illness.[113] Known as "parasyphilis," this phase of the infection was characterized by two conditions: locomotor ataxia (characterized by a shifting, unsteady gait, also known as tabes) and paresis (also known as general paralysis of the insane). According to the consensus view, black patients only rarely fell prey to parasyphilis. Explaining this, doctors argued that symptoms like paresis were "limited to the brain of the civilized man"—that only those who were "exposed to the emotional stresses and strains of an active competitive life" could progress to this stage of the disease.[114] "Anyone who has seen a great many cases of tabes," observed one doctor,

> has perhaps noted that the subjects of this disease are for the most part drafted from a class of persons who work assiduously and get much friction of their lives; who feel the brunt of care and responsibility greatly, and who depress themselves with the tedium of their work and with apprehensive misgivings as to the possibility of failure, etc.; together with many other of the worries which rather seem to be the lot of the highly civilized white man. I am convinced that such temperamental and nervous defects have their influence in lowering the powers of resistance and in determining the development of tabes and the primary degenerative changes in the nervous system.[115]

African Americans, by contrast, were said to be "protect[ed]" from "the bad effect of severe emotions on the nervous system."[116] Being "very little liable to the serious disappointments of those in higher social stations," black men and women who contracted syphilis need not worry about suffering from paresis or tabes.[117] Something "native" to their organisms, it was believed, shielded them from "the distant nervous effects of syphilis."

The corollary of this was that for African Americans, syphilis was purely a disease of the body. When describing its symptoms, doctors fixated on outward, external manifestations, noting how black patients were more likely than white ones to develop "destructive" lesions, suppurations, and glandular enlargements.[118] Cutaneous scars were said to be "strikingly characteristic of the negro," not only "much more frequent" than in white patients but also "much more extensive."[119] According to one observer, syphilis in African Americans was "often quite precocious," as it was "not an uncommon thing" to see patients develop its earliest signs (bubo, chancre, eruption, mucous patches on the throat, fever, etc.) simultaneously, a phenomenon leading to "systemic infection and intoxication." As a result, "the entire cardio-vascular system becomes overwhelmed."[120]

In their treatment of black VD patients, doctors advocated for institutionalization, questioning "whether any black is ever efficiently treated except while confined in a hospital ward."[121] Within these settings, the preferred remedy was "constitutional medicine," which the infected "should be compelled to take."[122] Any attempt to teach African Americans the "laws of hygiene" doctors reasoned, was bound to fail; as one put it, "teaching [black patients] the hygiene of the disease" was "so hopeless that . . . it would be a farce were it not a tragedy."[123]

The reason for this speaks to the racial assumptions coloring doctors' perception of syphilis. What made black sufferers ineligible for hygienic therapy, quite simply, was their amorality. "The negro [syphilitic]," intoned one member of the medical profession, "does not feel the sense of shame and guilt which rises in the breast of the white man."[124] With most physicians believing that among African Americans, "adultery or fornication is literally not regarded as a sin," it seemed the only solution was "forced treatment under hospital care."[125] After all, if it was true that "negroes are practically without morals," then what hope was there for the kinds of personal reformation the hygienic treatment of syphilis aimed at?[126]

The healers of Hot Springs contributed to this racialized discourse. With the demise of the "civilized regime" that was slavery, one local doctor opined, syphilis had run rampant "among our negro population," as African Americans were "little better than animals with strong sexual passions."[127] Echoing this, a colleague pointed to "the negro's almost absolute lack of morality and cleanliness," arguing that it was "difficult to persuade the average negro . . . that sexual indulgence is wrong, even if he is in the actively infectious stage of syphilis."[128] Finally, like other white MDs, they concurred that the disease progressed differently in blacks and whites. As one local healer declared, though syphilis was "frequently encountered" among black southerners, "we do not recall the fact in our experience . . . of ever having seen a single case of tabetic disease in a negro."[129]

Beliefs such as these were widespread within Hot Springs and worked to limit the number of black health seekers at the resort. In keeping with the traditions of Jim Crow, the vast majority of the city's private hotels and bathhouses refused to admit African American visitors. After traveling to the resort, an organizer with the National Association of Colored Women observed that "because of a mere accident of our color," the members of her party "were forced to confine ourselves to an exterior observation of these bath palaces."[130] For their part, black newspapers discouraged readers from journeying into central Arkansas, noting that northern health resorts and spas were "more attractive than Hot Springs" on account of the latter's "awful . . . Jim Crow cars and other uncivilized offerings to the colored visitor."[131]

The realities of racial segregation and discrimination worked to confine most of the city's black health seekers to the free bathhouse the government ran. A typical experience here was that of Henry Fitzhugh, a black man who moved from Little Rock to Hot Springs in 1876 to be treated for rheumatism.[132] As he recalled decades later, before relocating, Fitzhugh was "down with it so bad the doctor had done give me up. He'd stopped giving me medicine. But the lady I was working for, she run a hotel in Poplar Bluff. They put me on a stretcher and they put me in the baggage car and they brought me clean on in to Hot Springs. They bathed me at the free bath house. I started feeling better right away. Twasn't long before I was well and able to work. I stayed right on here in Hot Springs."[133] After recovering, Fitzhugh opened a shoeshining establishment and made a success-ful living as a businessman until an injury forced him into retirement.

For African American visitors, there were only two alternatives to the govern-ment bathhouse: the Saint Pythias Sanitarium and the Crystal Bath Palace. Ac-cording to one early twentieth-century account, in the first few years after its opening, "thousands of colored people" benefited from "the scientific application of the waters" provided at Saint Pythias (also known as the Wade Infirmary).[134] Within these establishments, black doctors used many of the same curative meth-ods as the city's white medical men, and among their patients were those suf-fering from venereal disease. As a black physician named Harold Phipps ob-served, the elimination of "syphilitic poisons" was hastened by the city's hot baths, which allowed for the administration of "much larger doses of mercury . . . than would otherwise be possible."[135]

The extent to which doctors such as Wade or Phipps made use of hygienic therapies is unknown. While noting the value of "rest, rigid routine of treatment, [and] abstinence from alcohol and all forms of excitement" as a general medical principle, black healers published no material on this in connection with syphi-lis.[136] Nor do the reports of black syphilitics sent to Hot Springs by nonresident practitioners make mention of "hygienic treatment."[137] The city's white physicians also had little to say about black health seekers.[138] Knowing that their African

American counterparts also made use of the springs in conjunction with large doses of mercury, it is possible that they developed "hygienic treatment" to differentiate their curative methods from those used on black health seekers.[139]

Ironically, however, aspects of this form of therapy may have originated in African American curative responses to syphilis. On the whole, little is known about how infected black men and women dealt with this disease. White doctors who wanted to counter the "very prevalent" belief that "the negro race is all syphilitic" observed that "the negro who lives on good plain food, leads an out-door life, especially in the sun, avoids overindulgence in alcoholics, wisely avoids the iodides—in fact, neglects standard lines of medication—will, after one summer of sweat and sunshine, find himself with a sleek hide and all of his syphilis left behind."[140] Whites wishing to avoid the "disastrous sequelae" of syphilis, this writer advised, would be wise to emulate such habits.[141] Their similarities with the curative regimen practiced in Hot Springs suggests that the resort's white doctors might have been influenced by elements of black therapeutics. Given the fact that white southern MDs "borrowed freely from African American pharmacology" all across the region, such a possibility cannot be discounted.[142]

Among patients of their own race, white doctors showed great concern for "sexual excesses" and "morbid habits," believing that these had to be terminated.[143] Here, the emphasis was on "hygiene and the great moral principle of right," a fact reflecting doctors' faith in their white clientele's capacity for "personal reformation." As this indicates, hygienic therapy existed not only to heal diseased bodies but also to restore the privileged racial identities of Hot Springs' venereal health seekers.

For contemporary doctors, this was an imperative task. Venereal specialists connected the phenomenon of "race suicide" to purported increases in the prevalence of syphilis and gonorrhea, arguing that these diseases were "racial poisons" that exerted a degenerative force on the nation's germ plasm.[144] In order to secure the "future of the race," they argued, a variety of medical and public health measures would be required—including the banning of venereally infected immigrants, the screening of prospective spouses for syphilis and gonorrhea, and the sterilization of those deemed responsible for spreading these diseases.[145] Uplifting the moral standards of allegedly respectable, well-to-do syphilitic white men was a crucial part of this eugenic campaign, as without these individuals, the country would become the preserve of "inferior beings" unable to uphold America's standing in the world.[146] Civilization itself was at stake, and it was this fear that animated Hot Springs' response to syphilis. As one local practitioner put it: "We as a race are fast becoming a nation of syphilitics."[147] Only by reforming

the "perverted passions" of those who had grown up "denying themselves nothing that their sexual appetites demand" would this trend be reversed, and this
belief made moral therapy an essential part of Hot Springs' response to syphilis.

Syphilis, Rest Cure, and Race

It was not only through moral treatment that Hot Springs' white physicians severed hygienic therapy from its association with "amoral" African Americans.
While this strict regimen demanded that patients live in accordance with "the
great moral principle of right," other aspects of hygienic therapy were more compassionate. Among these was "rest cure"—a popular remedy for neurasthenia,
perhaps the era's foremost disease of civilization. Literally meaning "nervous exhaustion," neurasthenia was a condition thought to result from the breakneck
speed of "modern high-pressure civilization."[148] Its victims were largely "overworked business and professional men," whose overexposure to trains, steam-
ships, telegraphs, and the myriad other technological advances of an industrial
age left them mentally and physically crippled.[149]

A diagnosis laden with racist ideologies, neurasthenia was a quintessential
fin-de-siècle disease of middle- and upper-class whites. During the late nineteenth century, doctors gathered mounting evidence of the spread of insanity
and other adverse mental health conditions among the recently freed African
Americans of the US South. For many, this phenomenon was a worrying one,
especially given the fact that at the time, insanity was seen as a sign of intellectual progress. As historians have shown, so as to counter the notion that ex-
slaves were *progressing*, doctors drew a color line "right through the concept of
insanity."[150] Neurasthenia was central to this project; according to neurologist
George Beard, who did much to popularize the concept, Native Americans and
African Americans "suffer[ed] but little this way."[151] Indeed, whereas whites were
said to fall prey to insanity on account of the "pressures and responsibilities of
civilization," nonwhites did so because their minds were "unfit for civilization."[152] The latter diagnosis encouraged a punitive approach to insanity; the former, a more empathetic, compassionate one. In cases of neurasthenia, doctors
generally prescribed "rest cure," which necessitated withdrawal from daily work
routines and often from society itself.[153] Spas, baths, and health resorts were a
favored destination among the neurasthenic, who sought in these remote locations a gentle respite from the "evils of civilization."[154]

Hot Springs was one of these neurasthenic havens.[155] Especially with the resort's gentrification during the late nineteenth century, visitors to the area began
to remark on how its waters benefited the "nervously overworked" and how the

natural beauty of the Ozarks restored to health those suffering from "the great strain of our modern life with its increased mental activities."[156] Testifying to the resort's popularity among those diagnosed with neurasthenia, in 1892, a poem published in the pages of the *Hot Springs Medical Journal* offered a characterization of the typical health seeker:

His mind upset with business cares,
    And body much distressed,
The young man in Chicago pines
    For needed change and rest.

He grumbles at the early spring;
    With weather chill and raw,
Takes Doc's advice and starteth off
    To Hot Springs, Arkansaw.

He buys a ticket for the bath,
Of the Park Hotel becomes a guest,
Discards cigars for chewing gum,
    Goes in for change and rest.

One week gone by, he's all played out,
    His mind is sore depressed,
He finds the bathman has his change,
And the hotel has the rest.[157]

When coupled with "proper exercise and diet," doctors observed, bathing in and drinking the city's waters greatly benefited "fagged-out brain workers," who often returned from Hot Springs "sound and well."[158]

Resident healers perpetuated these notions, contending that the springs' therapeutic powers derived in part from "the *rest* from business duties" that could be secured here.[159] Coming from the "crowded and rushing life of the city," the typical health seeker found in Hot Springs

The exhilarating life of the pure country air, laden with all of the freshness of the Ozark Mountains—from the dust and hurry and strife of the busy city to the quietness and freshness and greenness of the forests to a home in the woods, practically, for the forests are all about him. Here he may spend, not only a few hours, but all of his days, under the shade of the trees. From business cares to absolute rest; from worry to peace; from the noise and dust and turmoil, if he wishes it, to a perpetual Sabbath. He may sit in the beautiful park on Hot Springs Mountain and see the world pass beneath him and be simply a looker-on.[160]

Touting rest as the "missing therapeutic agent" for patients whose nervous systems were "exhausted," resident doctors declared that the resort's "hot waters," "pure air," "picturesque location," and "freedom from business" had a "magical effect in bringing about relief to the patient."[161]

Local physicians were somewhat preoccupied by neurasthenia. Living and working at a place specializing in rest cure, they came to believe that a multitude of maladies could ultimately be traced back to "over-exertion," which "enfeebl[ed] the mind" and "reduced one's nervous energy."[162] Out of this neurasthenic discourse came new disease concepts like "mental rheumatism," a condition said to be common among "overworked" professionals who performed "great mental work for an unusual length of time, without rest or recreation."[163]

Similar themes colored local descriptions of VD. In an 1891 address to the Hot Springs Medical Society, for example, resident physician M. G. Thompson presented gonorrhea as a disease whose mental and emotional symptoms were often entirely neglected. This was particularly the case among patients forced to endure "butchery" and "mutilation" at the hands of physicians whose insistence on urethrotomies and perineal sections often left them without the powers of erection and ejaculation.[164] These surgical operations were injurious in a physical *and* psychological sense, Thompson argued, as patients subjected to them often experienced "depression and hysterical hallucinations making life almost intolerable."[165] The successful treatment of gonorrhea therefore required not only "therapeutic agents" but also a curative regimen designed to improve one's "mental condition." Hot Springs was the ideal place to implement such a therapeutic strategy: according to Thompson, the resort's "great advantage" in the treatment of VD owed to "the moral effect" the springs exerted on "the patient's mind."[166]

In promoting "rest cure," local healers also linked neurasthenia to syphilis. According to resident medical men, the typical syphilitic arrived in Hot Springs "wearied with life, tired . . . wearied with thought—wearied with cheer that is no comfort, with sleep that is no balm." "The wretched soul cursed with syphilis," one doctor explained, had

> From the time of the initial lesion learned to dread the sequels—he has spent his laid-up earnings seeking treatment that does not heal; his fears are growing; his physician implores him to be cheerful, and all will be well in time. He is alone in

his misery. He is ashamed; there is wasting of energy, of nerve power, of courage, of vitality. The long-hoped-for relief is not found. His confidence begins to wane; the physician is disappointed, disgusted and neglectful. His treatment has been eminently correct, and the result would have been perfect but for one indication which he can not meet—rest for the nervous system and rest for the mind.[167]

Local doctors believed that Hot Springs' "great advantage" in the treatment of syphilis lay in the effect the resort had on "the patient's mind."[168] Imagining the venereally afflicted health seeker as "the society man" or "the business man," they put forward a therapeutic program aimed at improving the health seekers' "mental condition"—at promoting "free[dom] from business cares" and relief from "overwork."

Ideas such as these had a tangible influence on medical practice within Hot Springs, which the case of one Joseph Cloidt offers evidence of. In 1911, Cloidt, a seventy-two-year-old ex-soldier, journeyed to Hot Springs on account of a "little spot" that had appeared on his penis. On two prior occasions, he had received treatment for VD, and after examining him, doctors acknowledged the "possible existence of syphilis." But instead of receiving a venereal diagnosis, Cloidt was informed that he had neurasthenia. "About the same time the patient developed the last lesion on his penis," his doctor observed, he had made "a bad business investment," which caused him to "worr[y] continually about his financial condition." As such, Cloidt's "little spot" was simply the product of "worry," of one's "physical and financial condition [being] constantly on [one's] mind."[169]

One year earlier, a Hot Springs physician named James Chesnutt encountered a patient suffering from many of the same symptoms. Over the course of the last few years, Chesnutt learned, this fifty-four-year-old man had become progressively "forgetful" and "inattentive to his business."[170] Though formerly a successful entrepreneur, all of his recent financial ventures had ended in failure, personal outcomes that—according to Chesnutt—indicated "failing mental power," "loss of memory," and general "lack of judgment."[171] Originally suspecting that he was suffering from neurasthenia, Chesnutt's diagnosis changed after this generally "dull and stupid" patient responded to one of his queries with the words "it is the third stage of syphilis."[172] After being placed on a lengthy course of mercurial inunctions and potassium iodide, the man made a remarkable recovery, gaining the "return of his mentality" and becoming "normal in all respects."[173]

Though the doctors in the two aforementioned cases reached opposing clinical conclusions in the diagnosis of their respective patients, their handling of

these unrelated cases exhibited one key commonality: the connection each practitioner made between syphilis and neurasthenia. Whereas the former diagnosed
neurasthenia in a man presenting some of the telltale signs of syphilis, the latter diagnosed syphilis in a man presenting some of the classic symptoms of neurasthenia. That these medical practitioners should so closely associate syphilis (a
disease typically associated with the poor, lowly, and immoral) with neurasthenia (a fashionable disease of the rich and respectable) may seem odd, as historical analyses have repeatedly demonstrated this venereal disease's cultural status
as a classic condition of the "other." Yet in turn-of-the-century Hot Springs, this
was not the case; here, doctors routinely identified syphilis as an affliction of the
affluent, responding to it with rest cure and "hygienic treatment" and in the process shearing this VD of its association with African Americans and other marginalized populations.

Conclusion

Local healers promoted the hygienic identity of syphilis in Hot Springs in order
to reduce the social stigma of VD among their largely middle- and upper-class
white patients. As their efforts demonstrate, hygienic treatment was about much
more than the physical care of the venereally afflicted. Syphilis in Hot Springs
was a cultural entity born of a particular set of understandings about race, sexuality, and class. The "hygienic" shape syphilis assumed at this central Arkansas
health resort was a consequence of doctors' and patients' attempts to sever this
venereal malady from its traditional associations with various marginalized
"others" and to shore up their patients' threatened identities in the process.[174]
Because it linked this venereal disease to a set of otherwise desirable qualities,
the "hygienic treatment of syphilis" accomplished these ends, enabling those
who journeyed to and resided within Hot Springs to uphold the cultural standing of the nation's dominant socioeconomic group.

The effects of this curative program were felt far outside Hot Springs. As the
resort's popularity grew, so too did that of its unique approach to syphilis. Many
of the doctors who visited the city around the turn of the century left convinced
that while the medicinal value of the springs was "nil," there was nevertheless
much to be learned from doctors' handling of syphilitic patients.[175] The methods
practiced here were those that *"should be practiced* by every practitioner," proclaimed one convert.[176] Visiting the resort showed this doctor that the cure of
syphilis entailed much more than the administration of drugs. "The treatment
must first of all be moral in character," he noted, adding that dietetic, hygienic,
and hydrotherapeutic measures were also necessary.[177] "By such methods," this

enthusiast declared, syphilitic patients would "gladly consent to stay at home," and moreover, would "see the results."[178]

Not all of those who adapted the Hot Springs treatment did so to prevent prospective patients from journeying to the city.[179] And some came away from their visits to Hot Springs having learned different lessons than others.[180] Nevertheless, the stimulus local doctors provided to venereology was impressive, and it reverberated across the nation. Through publishing articles, traveling to medical conferences, and speaking with visiting doctors, resort physicians gradually convinced colleagues of their professionalism and expertise.[181] They were "correct in what they said about many things," remarked one VD specialist after speaking with two Hot Springs physicians at a meeting in New Orleans.[182] Admissions such as these paved the road for the outward dissemination of antisyphilitic practices from the hinterland that was Hot Springs to the rest of the country.

Over the course of the 1910s, however, the "hygienic" approach to syphilis fell out of use at Hot Springs, as rest cure and moral treatment slowly gave way to a strictly water-based cure of this venereal malady. Yet despite this movement from hygiene to hydrotherapy, throughout the early twentieth century, racial theories continued to inform the diagnosis and treatment of syphilis at this central Arkansas resort. Moreover, with the passage of time, syphilis's identity here became ever more tightly yoked to the place that was Hot Springs. That this was the case is a surprising finding, especially given the remarkably *different* understanding of syphilis the medical profession wielded after 1905, when medical scientists isolated the disease's causative agent and subsequently devised an entirely new means of diagnosing and treating this venereal disorder. It is to these advances in medical technology, and to their impact on Hot Springs, that we now turn.

CHAPTER THREE

Diagnosing Syphilis at Army and Navy Hospital, 1890–1912

On June 11, 1911, Paul Jones entered the Hot Springs Army and Navy General Hospital complaining of back pain. A thirty-year-old army veteran, Jones had traveled to Hot Springs from Washington, DC, and shortly after being admitted, he was diagnosed with muscular rheumatism and placed on a regimen of baths, hot packs, and aspirin. This course of treatment brought a slight improvement to his condition, but after a few weeks in Hot Springs, Jones's lumbar discomfort persisted. At this point, hospital doctors began to suspect that his aches and pains were but the symptoms of a more serious, underlying malady. During his initial interview, Jones had admitted to contracting a venereal "bubo" some eight years earlier, and on the basis of this information, on July 16, the hospital's chief surgeon ordered a Wassermann test, sending a sample of his blood to Washington, DC, for laboratory analysis.

On July 24, the results of this test came back positive. That same day, Jones's doctors obtained a "further history" from their patient, who revealed that he had contracted syphilis "about seven years ago." This was followed by a general eruption, for which Jones took treatment. When his symptoms subsided, he stopped taking medicine. Upon learning of these additional details, hospital doctors diagnosed Jones with secondary syphilis, and gave him a combination of mercury, potassium iodide, and Salvarsan. These standard antisyphilitic treatments continued until August 17, when Jones—now feeling "much better"—left the hospital. Prior to this, a second blood sample was sent to Washington, DC, and on August 19, the results of this returned negative.[1]

Paul Jones's experience highlights many central developments in late nineteenth- and early twentieth-century Western medicine. With the advent of germ theory in the 1870s, European bacteriologists succeeded in isolating the causal agents of a number of deadly infectious diseases, including gonorrhea (1872), typhoid fever (1880), tuberculosis (1882), diphtheria (1882), cholera (1883), and bubonic plague (1894). For syphilis, the first decade of the twentieth century proved especially pivotal, as in quick succession, scientists discovered the disease's bacterial cause (*Treponema pallidum*, uncovered in 1905), developed a means for detecting its presence in the blood (the Wassermann reaction, 1906), and developed a more effective drug for treating it (Salvarsan, 1910).

Contemporary medical authorities often cast these innovations in revolutionary terms, crediting them with the wholesale overturning of established diagnostic and therapeutic methods. Speaking of the Wassermann test, for example, enthusiasts claimed that this new technology was of "inestimable value in the diagnosis of syphilis," that it would render the disease's detection "easy," and that it would "offer a definite means of determining the effectiveness of the treatment" of syphilis.[2] In their analyses of the early history of the Wassermann, scholars sometimes echo these sentiments, arguing that doctors viewed positive results as "infallible proof of treponemal infection."[3] Others contest the idea that diagnoses of syphilis were made solely on the basis of Wassermann test results, arguing instead that these were "never relied upon, alone, by wise physicians," as "clinical experience remained important."[4] According to the most recent study on the subject, many doctors used the Wassermann simply "to reinforce or adjust diagnostic and clinical decisions that had already been made using more traditional methods."[5] Beyond this, some historians contend that cultural ideologies factored into doctors' decisions about what was and what was not syphilis, as ideas of race and class made the diagnostic process an act of "social and moral assessment."[6] In her study of the Wassermann's use in early twentieth-century Scottish psychiatric facilities, for example, Gayle Davis finds that doctors more readily diagnosed the condition known as general paresis of the insane (GPI, a common complication of tertiary syphilis) in patients with histories of "excessive alcohol consumption" or "promiscuous sexual intercourse."[7]

These varied views on the Wassermann's significance are but a subset of a larger scholarly debate over how "revolutionary" turn-of-the-century medical technologies like this serological test were.[8] To date, this debate has been conducted largely via reference to published literature—including medical journals, books, and various governmental records. While important, these sources reveal little about the day-to-day *practice* of medicine; they cannot therefore speak to important questions about how doctors actually used (or did not use) the era's new diagnostic devices. Patient case files, on the other hand, offer an opportunity to do just that— that is, to see to what degree physicians adopted the era's novel means for detecting disease and to determine how they made sense of the data produced from these.

As a recent study of its early history correctly observes, the Wassermann "could only become a clinically usable test because serologists set out to actively engage clinicians, address their diagnostic and therapeutic interests and enrol them into cooperative ventures."[9] So, how was the Wassermann made into a "clinically usable test"? Under what circumstances did doctors call upon this new technology? To what extent did it influence their diagnostic and therapeutic decisions? And what does this tell us about the "laboratory revolution"?

As the case of Paul Jones reveals, the emergence of the Wassermann test did *not* prompt physicians to jettison more traditional approaches to diagnosis. At first glance, it might appear that they did, for the results of Jones's test helped doctors correctly identify the syphilitic cause of his rheumatism. However, consider two facts: hospital physicians only decided to send a sample of Jones's blood for testing *after* learning that he had suffered a venereal sore eight years prior to his trip to Hot Springs, and hospital physicians only decided to treat Jones for syphilis *after* extracting additional information from him, during which he admitted to taking medicines for syphilis sometime after this sore appeared. In other words, both the decision to administer a Wassermann and to trust its results were prompted by patient testimony—that is, by the detailed taking of a case history based on subjective evidence provided by Jones. In the end, it was this traditional method that drove doctors' decision to diagnose Jones with a venereal infection, not the Wassermann test.

Jones's experience was not unique. Indeed, it was rather representative of the Wassermann's more general implementation at the Hot Springs Army and Navy General Hospital. First made available to physicians in 1910, the test quickly became an accepted part of the facility's antivenereal efforts. Yet as an analysis of the hospital's clinical case files reveals, instead of holding it up as a source of "infallible proof," doctors looked on the Wassermann with a modicum of skepticism, refusing to award it pride of place within their diagnostic toolkits. This new technology was but an *aid* to diagnosis, occupying an auxiliary status far below doctors' preferred source of medical knowledge: patient testimony. Throughout the late nineteenth and early twentieth centuries, Army and Navy physicians regularly prioritized case histories over other diagnostic procedures, allowing soldiers' personal accounts to drive their understanding of VD. This was true both before and after the Wasserman's introduction and suggests that at least with regard to venereology, there was no "laboratory revolution" in turn-of-the-century medical practice.[10]

This is not to imply that nothing changed during the first few decades of the hospital's existence. Shortly after its opening in 1887, hospital administrators announced that syphilitic servicemen would be forbidden from receiving treatment here. Likely shaped by a mix of moral and monetary concerns, the VD ban had a rather unintended consequence: instead of keeping syphilis and gonorrhea out of the hospital, it limited doctors' access to patient testimony, as many applicants feared being turned away should knowledge of their venereal histories become known. Acknowledging that it only hampered doctors' ability to accurately diagnose cases of syphilis, in 1910, Army and Navy terminated this policy. In response, patients became more willing to discuss their sex lives, and correspondingly, doctors became much more confident in their pronouncements of syphilis. Importantly, it was this policy shift, not the introduction of the Wassermann test, that improved doctors' diagnostic capabilities.

Moreover, it should be noted that before 1910, patients' general reluctance to divulge the details of their sexual histories owed to practical concerns rather than moral ones. Interestingly, even during the period of the venereal ban, some patients' testimonies were remarkably honest, although the majority denied any prior contraction of syphilis or gonorrhea. That their statements became more candid after 1910 owed neither to an increase of syphilis among the general population nor to the destigmatization of American attitudes toward VD. Throughout the early twentieth century, notions of shame and guilt continued to infuse the country's venereal discourse. But this had little impact at Army and Navy, either with respect to sufferers or healers—who generally refrained from acting on whatever misgivings they might have harbored in connection with patients' personal conduct. Thus, the history of Army and Navy's experience with VD shows that American responses to syphilis were informed by many other elements besides morality.

The Creation of Hot Springs Army and Navy Hospital

Hot Springs Army and Navy General Hospital opened on January 17, 1887. The first permanent general hospital created by the US military, Army and Navy came into existence at a time of sweeping changes to the nation's medical infrastructure. Prior to the Civil War, hospitals were rather few in number and existed generally as charitable institutions for the poor and needy. Between 1873 and 1909, however, the number of hospitals in the country increased from 178 to over 4,300, as improvements in sanitation and medical technology—along with the emergence of more secular, scientific ideas about disease—combined to transform this singular institution into the primary site of medical treatment.[11] These developments, along with the incipient nationalism of the Progressive Era, the country's growing imperial ambitions, increasing public acceptance of the notion of a peacetime army, and a growing number of Civil War veterans seeking pensions and stipends, helped convince military leaders that existing systems of emergency care were no longer sufficient to meet the needs of a modern army and navy.[12] Designed to meet the long-term care needs of current and former servicemen, Hot Springs Army and Navy General Hospital was but one of three centralized, all-purpose medical institutions created by the federal government during this period.[13] The other two were the Army General Hospital at Washington Barracks in Washington, DC (renamed Walter Reed Hospital in 1909) and the General Hospital in San Francisco (renamed the Letterman Hospital in 1911).[14] In 1899 the government also created a special tuberculosis hospital for soldiers in Fort Bayard, New Mexico.[15] With these institutions in place, the stage was set for the modernization of American military health care.

As the US military expanded its health care apparatus, VD assumed increasing importance. In part, this trend reflected growing anxieties over syphilis and gonorrhea within American society more generally, but concerns over the country's capacity to function as a colonial power also contributed to it. Throughout this period, military leaders nervously fretted over the incidence of syphilis and gonorrhea within the various branches of the armed forces, diseases whose incidence in the aftermath of the Spanish-American War seemed to be rapidly increasing.[16] Confronting the specter of a military greatly diminished in strength owing to sicknesses of a venereal origin, army and navy commanders instituted a wide range of policies aimed at stopping the spread of sexually transmitted disease—the most controversial of which was an attempt to introduce a system of regulated prostitution into the Philippine Islands.[17] Though this particular disease-control measure proved to be rather short lived, the military's increased attention to syphilis and gonorrhea also manifested itself in the distribution of prophylactic kits to servicemen and the establishment of venereal wards within its overseas hospitals.[18] Within the United States, the general hospitals in San Francisco and Washington, DC, opened their doors to the victims of syphilis and gonorrhea as part of an attempt to reduce the military's crushing venereal burden.

As originally conceived, Hot Springs Army and Navy General Hospital was to be part of this mission as well. When it opened in January 1887, American military officials envisioned Army and Navy as a place where surgeons would specialize in the treatment of "such diseases as the waters of Hot Springs have an established reputation in benefiting."[19] This included syphilis. In 1887, the surgeon general informed military officials that "relief" of several conditions "traceable to specific infection" could be "reasonably expected from the use of the Hot

Springs waters."[20] An official report published the following year revealed that "a few" of the cases of rheumatism treated at Army and Navy were "found to be aggravated, if not induced, by a syphilitic taint," adding that "these specific cases were much benefited by the baths, combined with mercurial treatment."[21] Professional medical journals also recorded cases of soldiers being treated at the hospital for their "exposures and indiscretions."[22]

For some military officials, however, such a state of affairs was troubling. Believing that the acceptance of venereal cases attached a certain "odium" to the hospital, these voices soon became ascendant, and in the 1890s, a new policy appeared. Henceforth, Army and Navy would treat every illness the city's waters had "an established reputation in benefiting, *except that cases of venereal disease will not be admitted.*"[23] Military circulars warned base commanders across the country that "the transfer of venereal cases to the Army and Navy General Hospital, Arkansas, is prohibited" and that "in order that patients suffering from venereal diseases may not be permitted to enter this hospital," medical officers were to exercise "great care" when examining potential transfer cases to Hot Springs.[24] Military medical officers took this regulation seriously, often appending notes to the case files of soldiers transferred to Hot Springs certifying that they found "no evidence of any syphilitic or venereal disease."[25] Within Army and Navy, officials aimed to keep syphilitics from occupying hospital beds by adding a new section to the intake forms completed for all prospective patients. Entitled "venereal history," this required doctors to inspect all applicants for syphilis and to inquire about any prior instances of sexually transmitted illness. Those found to be infected would be turned away.

The reasons for this policy shift are not entirely clear. Very likely, considerations both moral and monetary played a role. With regard to the latter, it bears noting that the vast majority of Army and Navy's clientele were veterans of the Civil War, who received regular stipends for illnesses and injuries incurred in the line of duty. Technically speaking, these benefits were off limits to those suffering from syphilis (which was very much a disease *not* incurred in the line of duty). In reality, however, doctors often struggled to determine whether the symptoms of diseases like rheumatism, locomotor ataxia, and general paresis were venereal or nonvenereal origin and so sometimes awarded stipends to individuals suspected of having syphilis.[26] Given this, federal administrators likely reasoned that the only way to prevent these ex-soldiers from draining the military's financial resources (at a time when antivenereal expenses for *current* servicemen were already consuming much of the annual medical budget) was to preclude the entrance of syphilitic patients.

The belief that VD constituted the "wages of sin" likely fueled these arguments. Among those who criticized the hospital's venereal ban was W. F. Arnold, a navy surgeon. For Arnold, the government's decision to close Army and Navy to syphilitic servicemen was shameful, as it derived from the "theological deduction that venereal diseases are punishments for illicit sexual incontinence." The institution's refusal to treat them, he claimed, flowed out of the stigma surrounding syphilis and gonorrhea in American society, and he predicted that Army and Navy's calling attention to this stigma would force many prospective patients "to misrepresent the source of disabilities that really are venereal, in order to obtain admittance there."[27] His remarks are generally borne out by the hospital's clinical case files.

Syphilis at Army and Navy, 1887–1910

On the face of things, it seems that Army and Navy doctors upheld the hospital's proscription against venereal cases. For example, when in the summer of 1908 a soldier named Coleman McGray entered Army and Navy and promptly informed doctors that he had been taking treatment for a venereal sore contracted some eight months earlier, his request for care was rejected, and the words "NOT ADMITTED" were scrawled on his case file (box 35). Between 1887 and 1910, McGray was one of many men whose clinical records concluded with statements like "discharged for chronic gonorrhea," "discharged . . . for chancroids of the penis," and "discharged for constitutional syphilis in the secondary stage . . . not in line of duty."[28]

Interestingly, however, this was *not* the fate of every person who entered the hospital with a venereal illness. For every Coleman McGray turned away from Army and Navy, there were scores more men given "special permission" to enter the hospital and receive treatment for syphilis and/or gonorrhea.[29] Table 3.1 presents a simple statistical analysis of 2,173 patients treated at Army and Navy between 1898 and 1912. Though the hospital's annual reports make little mention of VD, its clinical records reveal that roughly 2 percent of all servicemen received a diagnosis of syphilis or gonorrhea. Official restrictions notwithstanding, Army and Navy did admit and treat the venereally afflicted.[30]

Among those treated for syphilis before the Wassermann's introduction in 1910 was Quinn Hawkins. A twenty-five-year-old private transferred to Army and Navy from Fort Riley, Kansas, Hawkins arrived in Hot Springs in the autumn of 1908 complaining of "soreness and stiffness" in the hips, knees, and ankle joints. Inquiring into his medical history, doctors learned that three years earlier, Hawkins had contracted a penile sore (for which he had taken "internal treatment").

TABLE 3.1

VD Diagnoses at the Hot Springs Army and Navy
General Hospital, 1898–1912

Box no.	Total no. of cases	No. of VD diagnoses
17	123	2
18	104	1
19	104	2
20	100	2
21	90	1
22	113	3
23	98	2
24	83	3
25	86	2
26	124	1
27	107	1
28	111	4
29	64	2
30	106	0
31	108	2
32	124	4
33	100	1
34	112	2
35	121	2
36	107	1
37	88	6
Totals	2,173	44

After reading his transfer card, which indicated not only that he "claims to have had syphilis" but also that he "feign[ed] rheumatism," a resident military surgeon diagnosed Hawkins with "tertiary syphilis." After three months' treatment with mercury and potash, he was returned to active duty (box 24).

As Hawkins's experience shows, Army and Navy *did* treat patients with VD—official rules to the contrary notwithstanding. And interestingly, despite these rules, like Hawkins, a fair proportion of patients answered doctors' venereal inquiries rather straightforwardly. When asked about his sexual history, one patient explained that he "noticed a sore yesterday" on his penis, adding that he "was with [a] woman seven days ago" (box 44). While some volunteered information of this sort in the hopes that it would facilitate recovery of health, others did so even knowing it had little to do with their present condition. Upon admittance, one patient revealed that he "had intercourse on average of six to eight times a year," while noting that he had never had any "symptoms relating to sexual intercourse" (box 44). Another freely discussed a "sore on [the] penis" that had appeared a year earlier, even though his illness pertained to a swollen right wrist (box 44). As this suggests, for some individuals, syphilis's status as the "wages of sin" led neither to feelings of shame and guilt nor to attempts at denial and concealment.

In their diagnostic efforts, doctors attached great importance to these personal testimonies. Consider the case of George Monday. After arriving in Hot Springs in the autumn of 1908, Monday complained of an ulcer that burst open when "the warm weather comes on." Upon admitting him into their care, hospital physicians initially diagnosed Monday with a simple case of eczema, for which they prescribed a homegrown compound called Ouachita oil. However, nearly one month into his stay in Hot Springs, doctors revised this assessment, modifying Monday's diagnosis to tertiary syphilis and placing him upon a regimen of mercury and potash. What triggered this reversal was Monday's open and honest venereal confession: in addition to admitting that he had previously suffered from gonorrhea, he explained that some four weeks prior to arriving in Hot Springs, he had contracted a sore on his penis. Such information led hospital physicians to conclude that the ulcer on his leg was *not* a sign of eczema, but of syphilis. Three weeks later, Monday returned home in an "improved" state of health (box 38).[31]

Army and Navy doctors were not alone in attributing such importance to the case history. Within turn-of-the-century medical circles, patient testimony was regarded as an indispensable aid to accurate venereal diagnosis. Having discovered that syphilis and gonorrhea were often the cause of conditions as varied as infant blindness, infertility, insanity, and locomotor ataxia, venereologists urged their colleagues toward a "more careful scrutiny" of their patients' sex lives, arguing that "too much emphasis cannot possibly be laid upon the obtaining of an accurate genito-urinary history."[32] Such a stance challenged the conventional wisdom that "all syphilitics are liars"—that is, that on account of things like "shame and family pride," individuals with a venereal disease invariably displayed a "tendency to concealment" when asked about the source of their medical troubles.[33] Without discounting it, specialists sought ways of working around this tendency; as one proposed, instead of asking "Have you ever had syphilis?" it was better to ask "When did you contract syphilis?"[34] Regardless of the tactic adopted, the message was clear: as "the civilized world is rapidly becoming syphilized," it was of the utmost importance to "inquire searchingly of the sexual life of our patients."[35]

Of course, case histories were not always necessary. At times, physical examination was sufficient to reveal a case of syphilis. For example, during the spring of 1908, hospital physicians diagnosed infantryman Adam Lepphardt with tertiary syphilis on the basis of his "slightly enlarged" glands, an "eruption" on the right leg, and numerous "small papulae" on his penis. For two months, Lepphardt received a steady diet of mercury and the iodides of potassium—his denial of any VD history notwithstanding (box 33). Doctors here felt themselves absolutely certain as to the venereal nature of Lepphardt's illness, as they did with a number of other patients displaying more or less obvious symptoms of syphilis.[36] But textbook cases like these were relatively rare. Often, the syphilitic underpinnings of a patient's problems only became clear after several months of failed treatment or only after repeat visits to Hot Springs.[37] For many others, uncertainty reigned.

That this was the case owed partially to the fact that many of the venereally afflicted soldiers and sailors who traveled to this health care facility around the turn of the century harbored old syphilitic infections, conditions that had progressed into the chronic ailments characteristic of the disease's tertiary stage. When faced with cases like these, doctors placed an especially high premium on autobiographical information. In this late stage of the disease, during which infection spreads to the cardiovascular and/or neurological systems, sufferers were often "entirely free from the gross or visible external manifestations of the disease."[38] Syphilis's characteristic skin lesions were "often wholly absent," and the bacteria that cause the disease were notoriously difficult to detect—even with advanced laboratory devices like the Wassermann test.[39] Given these obstacles, venereologists were particularly insistent on anamnesis when managing patients they suspected were in the final stage of the disease, arguing that "in making the diagnosis of tertiary syphilis, first the history of the patient is of importance."[40] "If a positive history of syphilis is obtainable," one authority declared, it would be of "some value in determining the character of a probable tertiary lesion."[41]

It is for this reason that local doctors placed a premium on patient testimony. So convinced of its value were hospital physicians that at times they allowed this to shape their diagnostic conclusions even when physical evidence pointed in a different direction. In this category belongs the case of Charles Gaffield, a sixty-one-year-old ex-regular who entered Army and Navy on April 29, 1904. When asked about his venereal history, Gaffield claimed that at the age of fourteen he had contracted syphilis after "trad[ing] drawers with a sailor," a statement that clearly befuddled the Canadian-born man's doctors, who observed that their patient was in "excellent" condition—his "pretended air of illness" notwithstanding. Concluding that Gaffield was "stupid and bent on playing the hypochondriac," Army and Navy surgeons nonetheless placed this military veteran on a course of mercury and other "specific" measures, evidently determining that on the basis of his positive history the "scars of erosive ulcers" they detected on his penis constituted an indication of "constitutional syphilis." Later that summer, Gaffield left Army and Navy, but the records we have do not comment on the status of his evidently "pretended" illness (box 19).

More common were the experiences of James McNeal and Walter Miller, two army veterans treated for syphilis in Hot Springs prior to the Wassermann's introduction. In both cases, physical difficulties prevented doctors from obtaining patient testimonies, which clearly complicated their diagnostic efforts. Attesting to the importance attached to history taking, a doctor declared in McNeal's case that "this man is very deaf and it is hard to get a clear history, but there is little doubt that he has constitutional syphilis." As these words indicate, the fact that resident physicians felt themselves able to definitively diagnose McNeal's condition *in spite of* their patient's hearing impairment reveals how much stock the institution put into the subjective data relayed to them by patients (box 37).

When he came to Army and Navy on April 3, 1909, Walter Miller was an immediate source of worry and diagnostic consternation to hospital physicians, who found themselves unable to obtain a "definite" venereal history from their patient "on account of aphasia." Although they detected "scars" on the under surface of Miller's penis, resident surgeons reported that they could not "get history of secondaries." Only after Miller's mother—who had accompanied him to Hot Springs in anticipation of such a difficulty—filled in the gaps in doctors' understanding did Army and Navy place their patient on a course of antisyphilitic remedies (box 37).

Cases such as these, admittedly, were rare. Although Army and Navy patients at times obliged their doctors' wishes for frankness, most men revealed little about their sexual histories.[42] When confronted with patients who "denied absolutely [any] sore on [the] penis" and who also showed inconclusive bodily evidence of syphilis, how did doctors decide whether a given illness was venereal in nature?[43] Given its status as the "wages of sin," one might expect behavioral clues to play a prominent role in this process, as evidence of immoral conduct such as excessive drinking, smoking, or sexual activity could, at least in difficult cases, tip the scales in favor of a venereal diagnosis. Interestingly, however, for neither McNeal nor Miller was this true: the first man received treatment for constitutional syphilis even though he admitted to nothing more than an occasional cigar; the second was put on a course of mercury inunctions in spite of the fact he showed no evidence of alcoholism or tobacco use. For these cases, social attitudes toward syphilis do not appear to have factored into clinical practice very significantly.

This was not always the case. At times, the diagnosis of VD was a social process, one informed by an assessment of a patient's moral status. This may have been true for Julius Hansen, a twenty-nine-year-old white private who came to Army and Navy on August 2, 1902. Upon admission, Hansen displayed a swollen right wrist, knee, and ankle; according to him, these symptoms constituted the lingering remnants of a malarial infection he had contracted in the Philippines. While agreeing that Hansen was suffering from rheumatism, hospital staff believed this had been aggravated by the man's "vicious habits"—including his tendency to "drink to excess" and his "connection with a woman" shortly before entering Hot Springs that he admitted to. Judging that Hansen was a man of "bad habits" and finding some evidence of a syphilitic infection, doctors ruled that his rheumatism was likely "venereal in origin" and so applied a solution of mercury bichloride to his penis (box 22).

On the whole, cases like these were extremely rare. Generally speaking, hospital staff refrained from acting on the perceived moral improprieties of their patients. A rather common experience was that of Lester Rhodes, who arrived at Army and Navy on May 30, 1910, with pains in the knees and ankles. Claiming "no history of venereal disease," Rhodes averred that his symptoms were the result of having been "thrown from a horse." Suspicious of this explanation and knowing that he sometimes drank "to excess," Rhodes's doctor observed that "from the character of the [venereal] denial it is believed patient is not telling the truth." Physical examination revealed "thickened places" in his urethra, and this prompted hospital staff to consider that Rhodes's ailment was "probably of gonorrheal origin." Despite this belief, however, doctors proceeded cautiously, treating their patient with a series of nonvenereal remedies. Even though doctors regarded him as untrustworthy, this influenced neither the diagnosis nor the treatment Rhodes received (box 44).[44]

Hospital staff also had good grounds for doubting the claims of James Mayo. Admitted to Army and Navy on February 18, 1906, Mayo sought treatment for joint pain and general feelings of bodily weakness. Upon examining him, doctors detected "multiple sores on the penis," which according to Mayo were the symptoms of "dhobie itch"—a tropical malady evidently contracted in the Philippines. Sensing subterfuge, an attending surgeon labeled Mayo "a suspect." Still, there was "no positive evidence that he has syphilis." At this point, doctors might have relied on what they knew of their patient's personal habits to resolve their diagnostic doubts. Doing so might have prompted them to declare his a case of syphilis, as Mayo admitted to "moderate" alcohol use, to having "smoked and chewed" tobacco for ten years, and to having contracted gonorrhea earlier in life. However, they did not do so; despite this information, Mayo's condition was diagnosed as articular rheumatism, and at no point during his hospital stay did he receive any antivenereal treatment (box 35).[45]

In cases involving black patients, however, doctors appear to have been less trusting. Though black soldiers only rarely entered Army and Navy, available evidence suggests that racism did impact clinical practice here. Such was certainly the case for Ed Grundy, a twenty-four-year-old black private admitted to the hospital on August 10, 1912, for "what he called neuralgia." As this statement indicates, from the very beginning of his stay, hospital personnel distrusted Grundy's statements; at one point, a doctor wrote that there was "a strong possibility of malingering in this case." After finding an ulcer inside his nose, Grundy's diagnosis was changed to tertiary syphilis, even though he denied having ever contracted this disease. On September 29, 1912, treatment with Salvarsan began, and this continued until October 10, when Grundy was returned to his home in Little Rock, his condition "improved" (box 22).

Elliott Hamp's experience at Army and Navy was fairly similar. A twenty-four-year-old black man who served as a private in the Tenth Cavalry, Hamp came to Hot Springs from Ft. Riley, Kansas, on January 17, 1909. Like many patients, Hamp complained of joint and muscle pains, along with headaches and "some vertigo." Neither physical examination nor patient testimony yielded much evidence of venereal infection. Nevertheless, his condition was diagnosed as tertiary syphilis. As his doctor explained in a letter to his commander at Ft. Riley dated March 9, 1909, Hamp "was treated with mercurial inunctions and increasing doses of potassium iodide." Claiming that this had yielded "marked beneficial results," his doctor recommended that antisyphilitic treatment be "continued" at Ft. Riley (box 23).

Another black patient admitted to Army and Navy was Samuel Jacobs. Said to be a man of "good" habits with "no history of VD," Jacobs arrived in Hot Springs on July 10, 1903, from Ft. Mackenzie, Wyoming, where he had been treated for articular rheumatism "without any apparent improvement in his condition." After inquiring into his history, doctors learned that Jacobs might have contracted a "chancre" in 1896 but initially agreed with the diagnosis previously given him. However, after weeks of "no change" in his condition, he was eventually given a "mercury shirt" and placed on inunction therapy. This antisyphilitic regimen continued for exactly one week, at which point a doctor scribbled the phrase "discontinue Hg" on his progress sheet. Shortly after this, Jacobs left the hospital, his condition unimproved, his body likely still feeling the effects of antisyphilitic medications administered in the absence of clear physical evidence of a venereal condition (box 29).

While it is unclear whether Jacobs's experience was typical of black patients, his case speaks to an additional strategy doctors sometimes relied on to resolve their diagnostic uncertainties: the "therapeutic test." In clinics and hospitals all across the United States, doctors sometimes experimented with mercury and other antivenereal compounds in cases suggestive of syphilis. Patients "without the classical initial lesion" and who "denie[d] or conceal[ed] a history of possible infection" were especially likely to be subjected to the therapeutic test.[46] According to its proponents, the procedure was of tremendous value, as even practitioners possessed of "the greatest skill and experience" could be "baffled" by syphilis, and "especially by the latter manifestations of the disease."[47]

Army and Navy physicians occasionally availed themselves of this method. Their use of it challenges the rather optimistic assessments of its benefits and suggests that it often led to disastrous results. Such was the case for T. O. Hutson, a forty-two-year-old contract surgeon who entered Hot Springs in August 1907. Shortly after being admitted, Hutson began displaying a number of profoundly disturbing symptoms, including a "melancholic temperament" and certain "suicidal tendencies." At one point he "point[ed] [a] loaded revolver at [his] chest." Because he also "had difficulty walking and in balancing himself," doctors wondered whether he had paraplegia ataxia, inserting a question mark after naming this as a possibility, which indicated an ambiguous diagnosis reflecting a suspicion of syphilis. Still, as he denied all evidence of a past or present venereal illness, doctors resisted the urge to act on these suspicions, at least until early October, when—three months after his admittance to the hospital—Hutson was placed on a course of mercurial inunctions. A little more than a month later, a doctor scribbled the order to "stop inunctions[,] . . . stop K.I.," and shortly after this, Hutson left the hospital, his condition "deteriorated" (box 27).[48]

T. O. Hutson was not the only Army and Navy patient subjected to the therapeutic test.[49] Nor was he the only serviceman whose progress sheet concluded with orders such as "omit Hg" or "stop mercury!"[50] Yet because of the inherent dangers toxic chemicals like mercury pose to the human body, such procedures were far from standard at the hospital. More often than not, doctors restrained themselves from giving antivenereal remedies to patients without a clear diagnosis, and even when syphilis was strongly suspected. Diagnostic uncertainty typically led to therapeutic inaction.

Such was the case for William Hoover. A twenty-four-year-old private from Ohio, Hoover arrived at Army and Navy in the spring of 1908. During his initial examination, Hoover presented several physical signs characteristic of a venereal illness, including a "marked general enlargement" of the glands. However, as Hoover insisted that he had "no history of venereal diseases" his doctors could do no better than offer a questioning diagnosis of syphilis. Six months later, Hoover left Army and Navy, his progress sheet failing to note any significant improvements (box 26).

Unresolved venereal suspicions also marked the case of James A. Huycke. A Kansas veteran in his early twenties, Huycke first arrived at Army and Navy on January 2, 1904. Upon inspection, doctors observed that his glands were "indurated and enlarged"; this symptom, along with a "suspicious thinness of the hair," led them toward an ambivalent diagnosis: "chronic muscular rheumatism, general (specific?)." Leaving the hospital without any change in his condition, Huycke returned the following March and then again in the spring of 1906. During his final visit, the man presented "brown spots" all over his body. When viewed in conjunction with the aforementioned symptoms, which persisted, Army and Navy surgeons rendered another conflicted verdict. "The case is extremely suspicious . . . of syphilitic infection," they concluded, "but at the same time there is nothing definite on which admission to the hospital can be denied." Therefore, as on his previous visits, hospital surgeons treated Huycke with nonvenereal remedies; despite his lack of improvement, no mercury or iodides of potassium ever entered his system (box 27).

The same was true for Russell Finney. Admitted on August 15, 1906, this ex-volunteer traveled to Hot Springs suffering from vertigo, insomnia, and ringing in the ears. Six weeks into his stay at Army and Navy, doctors noted that while he was "much improved," Finney's health remained suboptimal. Their suspicion was that these were likely the product of an untreated venereal infection. "It is most probable," a physician wrote, "that this is a case of tertiary syphilis, but the evidence is not sufficient to render an absolute diagnosis." On account of this uncertainty, Finney's treatment included neither mercury nor the iodides of potassium (box 17).

Cases like Hoover's, Huycke's, and Finney's were the norm at Army and Navy during the period of the venereal ban. Repeatedly wracked by indecision, hospital physicians regularly allowed patient testimony to guide their diagnostic and therapeutic decisions—even when their charges "showed all indication of being syphilitic."[51] Army and Navy's venereal ban resulted in the creation of a documentary record peppered with phrases such as "strongly suggestive of the eruption of syphilis," "suggests a specific infection," and "looks like syphilitic ulcers" and led to patients often receiving a series of nonvenereal medications that failed to alleviate their suffering. Between 1887 and 1910, it seems doctors were simply unable to tell what was a case of syphilis from what was not, frequently lamenting how—to cite one example—"from the history, physical examination, etc., [we] would say that this man is syphilitic, but there is no positive evidence" (box 33).

Statements such as these were an outgrowth of the hospital's venereal ban. Prior to 1910, individuals whose illnesses doctors regarded as being "probably specific" received diagnoses such as "syphilis secondary?," "tabes dorsalis (con-stitutional?)" "chronic articular rheumatism (probably specific)," "muscular rheu-matism (specific?)," and "chronic constipation (lues?)," and the like.[52] The prod-uct largely of negative VD testimonies, these ambivalent diagnoses were an outgrowth not of shameful attitudes toward syphilis but instead of Army and Navy's ban on the treatment of venereal cases. That something other than inter-nalized stigma drove the content of Army and Navy patients' personal histories can be seen through a comparison of them with venereal patients at another major military institution: the San Francisco General Hospital.

Syphilis at the San Francisco General Hospital, 1898–1912

In part, the difficulties Army and Navy doctors experienced diagnosing syphilis were universal and owed to the disease's rather protean, mysterious qualities. At clinics, hospitals, and doctors' offices all across the country, physicians struggled to distinguish syphilis from the many nonvenereal conditions whose symptoms it often overlapped with.[53] As even seasoned venereologists admitted, syphilis's seemingly infinite powers of metamorphosis made it a "most difficult" malady to detect; according to one specialist, "the man who would be a perfect syphilog-rapher needs to know everything to be known in medicine."[54]

Yet despite these general obstacles, the venereological confusion that reigned at Army and Navy was largely of the hospital's own making. A comparison with the General Hospital in San Francisco, which openly treated VD cases, reveals as much. On account of its lack of prohibitive measures, patients at the General Hos-pital were less circumspect about their sexual histories, and accordingly, doc-tors displayed none of the hesitation and diagnostic uncertainty seen in Hot Springs.

Because San Francisco General Hospital was unconcerned with screening out syphilis, its doctors were not asked to inquire into entrants' past encounters with VD. Resident physicians were, however, generally interested in the subject and often included any relevant information in a section of their case files entitled "personal history." In marked contrast to the patients at Army and Navy, patients at San Francisco General regularly spoke at some length about such episodes—even when they had little to do with their present complaint. Thus, whereas in Hot Springs, the most common term uttered with regard to VD was "denied," in San Francisco, patients reported "chancroids two months ago," "chancre last Feb-ruary," "thinks he might have had gonorrhea recently," "sore on penis about six years ago," and the like.[55]

Statements such as these went a long way toward curtailing the problem of diagnostic indecision. Consider the case of John Portwood. Admitted on November 8, 1906, Portwood presented a marked sciatica, complete with sharp pains along the left hip. While receiving treatment, doctors discovered a small abscess on the back of Portwood's left hand. Inquiring about this, they learned that about seven years earlier, their patient had a penile sore, which was "not followed by any of the signs of syphilis and for which he was never given antisyphilitic treatment." Because he displayed no other venereal symptoms, doctors noted that "there are only the histories of syphilis and gonorrhea to be mentioned as etiology factors." Despite this, Portwood was given potassium iodide for syphilis.[56]

A positive testimony also inclined Jason Race's doctors toward a diagnosis of syphilis. Entering the San Francisco hospital on November 11, 1906, Race reported muscle pains in his left leg and thigh. Upon examination, doctors found "faint scars" on the side of his penis, along with enlarged glands. Despite these signs, Race's initial diagnosis was chronic rheumatism. When treatment failed to improve his health, however, this was amended to syphilis. The reason? When he was admitted, Race provided the following VD history: "gonorrhea in 1901, cured in 1 month. Few months later had several small ulcers on penis (patient says 5 or 6 sores), cured in few weeks. . . . Doctor told patient he had soft chancres and gave him blood medicine for 3 months."[57]

Patients in San Francisco willingly provided doctors with extensive sexual histories even when their illnesses had nothing to do with VD. For example, when Henry O'Kinke entered the hospital on December 2, 1906, he immediately informed the resident surgeon that in April of the previous year, he had suffered from a "venereal ulcer," which doctors had variously pronounced as chancre or chancroid. For three months, O'Kinke received treatment for syphilis, and after this experienced "no secondaries." Despite the fact that he came to the hospital to be treated for tonsillitis, O'Kinke felt no qualms in confessing to earlier encounters with VD.[58]

What these cases suggest is that soldiers' reluctance to talk about VD did *not* derive primarily from feelings of shame. Had the denials so commonly uttered at Army and Navy stemmed from moral concerns, one suspects that negative testimonies would have surfaced with the same degree of regularity at the San Francisco hospital. That they did not means that something other than internalized stigma was determining the content of patients' personal histories. That something else was *policy*, a fact that becomes clear when we examine syphilis at Army and Navy after the Wassermann's introduction in 1910.

Syphilis at Army and Navy, 1910–1912

In the surgeon general's 1909 report, military leaders acknowledged the presence of a "large number of cases of syphilis in its secondary and tertiary manifestations" at Army and Navy. Also conceded was the "not uncommon inability of medical officers to recognize and properly treat these cases." Following the recommendation that it "relax" its prohibition on VD cases, the following year, military officials rescinded the hospital's ban, opening wide Army and Navy's doors to the nation's venereally afflicted servicemen.[59] In a matter of months, a policy that had been on the books for decades evaporated, and in relatively short order, Army and Navy acquired the status of a true "general hospital."[60]

This shift in policy created a new institutional environment within the hospital, one marked by less duplicitous doctor-patient relations. Typical of those admitted in this new era of candor was John Matkin. Immediately upon entering the hospital, Matkin informed resident doctors that he had received "three doses of 606 in 1911, the second being followed by a plus minus Wassermann." Admittedly "anxious to know the present condition of his blood following the 606 of last year," he made no attempt to disguise the fact that he had contracted syphilis; in deference to his wishes, hospital staff ordered a Wassermann test. Two weeks into his stay, this came back negative. Unfortunately, however, not long after this Matkin was dismissed from Army and Navy for traveling "downtown—where he "had a dose of Salvarsan given him" (box 35).

William Lewis also took advantage of the hospital's new policy in order to clear up his own syphilitic suspicions. Upon entering on August 1, 1912, Lewis immediately relayed to his doctors a recent venereal history: a primary sore in 1911, quickly followed by secondaries, for which he had taken "two injections of Salvarsan and six months of mercury." According to resident surgeons, Lewis's "chief complaint" was "a feeling of uncertainty with regard to syphilis." Like Matkin, what this twenty-three-year-old former seaman sought was a serological procedure, and when during his third week in Hot Springs Lewis's Wassermann test came back negative, hospital officials noted that this information "relieved him of much." Immediately after this, Lewis returned to his home in Hutchinson, Kansas (box 33). Similarly, after arriving at Army and Navy on May 1, 1911, Michael Pickard informed doctors that he "feared . . . his trouble might be luetic," though he was "quite certain" that he had never had "any initial lesion" (43).

As these cases demonstrate, once the hospital relaxed its policy toward syphilitics, patients became much more forthright about their sex lives. Instead of repeatedly recording the word "denied" on the venereal history section of their case files, doctors now filled these with lengthy accounts of patients' previous bouts with VD—with statements like "rheumatism has gotten much worse since contracting the gonorrhea six months ago," "gonorrhea eight years ago, rheumatism came on two months later," "the venereal attack was severe," and so on.[61] Armed with this information, doctors were able to quickly shed their diagnostic doubts and to replace them with a much more confident understanding of what was and was not a case of syphilis.

With this, diagnoses made on social and cultural grounds became even more infrequent than they had been prior to 1910. To be sure, hospital staff occasionally punished patients for moral infractions, such as one Clark Rainey. A thirty-seven-year- old private from Pennsylvania, Rainey entered the hospital on July 25, 1912. Like many others who came to Army and Navy after the lifting of the venereal ban, Rainey provided an extensive VD history: gonorrhea four years earlier, a hard chancre in January, 1911, and the symptoms of secondary syphilis shortly after that. Rainey also explained that he had received a "great deal of mercury" and two shots of Salvarsan, and on hearing of this, doctors sent a sample of his blood to Ft. Leavenworth for serological analysis. On August 5, the results of his Wassermann test came back negative. Having cleared this up and seeing that he presented "no active manifestations" of syphilis, doctors began treating Rainey for his other ailments—including a sore shoulder. On August 9, however, Rainey was discharged from the hospital for "drunken habits" (box 44).

Theodore Pilloud met a similar fate. A Swiss immigrant who first traveled to Hot Springs in 1908, Pilloud made a return trip in 1912, when he received a diagnosis of chronic lumbago. After a few weeks of treatment, he also developed a "most suspicious ulcer" in his throat. After questioning him, hospital staff learned that Pilloud had become accustomed to taking journeys in the mountains surrounding the city; on one of these outings, he was caught "accosting" several young girls. After his doctors learned of this, Pilloud was immediately discharged from the hospital, even though his ulcer had "not responded to local treatment" (box 43).

The case of Stephen Prouchard was similar. A seventy-two-year-old veteran from Canada, Prouchard arrived in Hot Springs on February 9, 1912, complaining of itching caused by a series of squamous eruptions on his legs and forearms. Though he admitted to contracting both syphilis and gonorrhea "forty-two years ago," doctors concluded that his illness was nonvenereal in origin and treated Prouchard for iritis. Early in his stay at Army and Navy, other patients regularly observed him in the lavatory "striking the head of his penis with his fingers." Hospital staff confirmed that Prouchard was undoubtedly a "chronic masturbator." Despite this, he received no punishment; after five months of treatment, he made "fair progress," and on July 15, Prouchard was sent home in an improved condition (box 44).

This was the extent of hospital staff's criticism of servicemen's personal habits. Receiving much more candid responses to their questions about patients' sex lives, doctors had little reason to doubt the veracity of their venereal testimonies, and this diminished opportunities for making diagnoses on moral grounds. The case of Charles Linninger further underscores this. Shortly after he entered Army and Navy in the autumn of 1911, physicians noted the presence of "many copper colored scars" across his body, in addition to a "general glandular induration." Had Linninger gone on to deny all evidence of past venereal infection, his attending surgeon would have likely rendered a diagnosis that left a hint of his unconfirmed venereal suspicion and then proceeded to experiment (or not) with antivenereal medications. But because of the hospital's policy reversal, Linninger confessed that he had "been taking mercury by mouth for the past eight months," on account of an earlier contracted venereal malady. After learning of this, hospital physicians placed their patient on a course of potassium iodide, their treatment of choice for "syphilis, tertiary" (box 32).

Perhaps the most interesting thing about Linninger's case is that he was not administered a Wassermann test. Introduced in 1910 (the same year officials repealed Army and Navy's ban on venereal cases), the new serological procedure rapidly became part of standard hospital practice. Despite this, it was *not* universally administered, and in fact, only half of all patients given a syphilitic diagnosis had blood samples sent away for this. Although it represented an important part of its diagnostic arsenal, within Army and Navy Hospital, the Wassermann was secondary to the case history.

In many cases, the new diagnostic tool was only called on when patient testimony pointed doctors in the direction of VD. This was true for Paul Jones (whose story is recounted in the beginning of this chapter) and also for Perry Fisher. Admitted to Army and Navy on May 30, 1912, Fisher came to Hot Springs complaining of "aches and pains in all bones." Initially diagnosed with chronic articular rheumatism and given a series of "cleansing baths," doctors began to consider the possibility of a venereal infection when this treatment failed to produce any notable improvement in his condition. What pushed them in this direction, despite the absence of physical symptoms, was the fact that Fisher had admitted to "gonorrhea in 1906" and "syphilis in 1905." He also connected these earlier problems to his current rheumatic troubles, reporting that "five years ago," he had "beg[un] to have pains in right ankle," and that he "had syphilis at that time also." Possessed of this knowledge, during his third week in Hot Springs hospital officials sent a sample of Fisher's blood to Washington, and when his Wassermann came back positive, this St. Louis native received an "additional diagnosis" of secondary syphilis, for which he was placed on a course of mercury and the iodides of potassium (box 12).[62]

As cases like Fisher's show, positive anamnesis often encouraged doctors to seek out serological confirmation of their syphilitic suspicions. But what if the results of this were negative? This was what happened to James C. Bowers, an ex-captain who arrived at the hospital on November 3, 1910. Although his transfer card stated that he was a victim of poliomyelitis, doctors suspected that Bowers's illness was venereal in nature, and as he had admitted to contracting syphilis some "twenty or thirty years ago," they officially diagnosed him with locomotor ataxia (a common complication of tertiary syphilis). Even though the Wassermann test they ordered for Bowers came back negative, doctors remained convinced of the source of his infirmities, and beginning in February of 1911 they treated him with "mercury inunctions and potassium iodide in large doses." Unfortunately, Bowers's illness had progressed to the point at which medicines could no longer be of benefit, and the following month doctors reported that their patient was "losing ground rapidly," with "great mental depression" (box 6). Despite this, hospital physicians did not waver in their venereal diagnosis.

That hospital doctors placed Bowers on a regimen of antisyphilitic drugs in spite of a negative Wassermann may have surprised those doctors who found case histories "a great source of error for the physician."[63] Yet as the aforementioned cases show, Army and Navy physicians did not believe that the Wassermann rendered the diagnosis of syphilis "easy." After 1910, resident medical men sought answers to their venereal questions using the same method they had prior to the Wassermann's appearance: through the taking of case histories. It was thus an old technique—the case history—that dictated how the Wassermann entered local medical practice.[64] Ultimately, it was this through traditional, clinical procedure that Army and Navy doctors aimed to unravel the secrets of syphilis.

If positive testimonies pushed doctors toward the Wassermann, it is also true that negative testimonies often pushed them away from it—even when physical examination aroused their own syphilitic suspicions! Such was the case for Charles Duffine, who throughout the winter of 1912 received treatment at Army and Navy for a condition diagnosed as "rheumatism." Upon examining him, hospital surgeons recorded a "strong suspicion of syphilis, tertiary," noting that while in the Philippine Islands, Duffine "was told he had lues." Yet "when inquiries began," he "began to evade, and refused a Wassermann," evidently because he was "afraid to have it on his record." As they observed no obvious signs of syphilis on his person, Duffine's medical attendants chose to accept the negative anamnesis he provided and placed him on a regimen containing neither mercury nor the iodides of potassium (box 15).[65]

Compared to Army and Navy, doctors at the Letterman Hospital made much greater use of the Wassermann test. Unlike in Hot Springs, where military practitioners typically only ordered serological testing if their patients' bodies or testimonies pointed toward syphilis, in San Francisco, the Wassermann was a routine part of the admissions process—often administered to soldiers within a day of their entrance to the hospital.[66] In addition to using this diagnostic device for servicemen whose symptoms betrayed no evidence of a venereal infection, Letterman Hospital physicians also placed greater faith in the results of Wassermann readings, treating patients with mercury and other antisyphilitic drugs even if the only evidence for this came in the form of a positive blood test.[67] The converse was true as well; those patients with evidence of syphilis but negative Wassermanns were generally kept off this class of medications.[68] Both practices diverged from the standards of clinical care followed at Army and Navy, where hospital physicians were much more circumspect in their interpretation and use of blood test results.

What explains this difference? In part, Army and Navy's comparatively lackluster faith in laboratory diagnostic methods likely came about as a result of their interactions with the resort's private practitioners, with whom they sometimes consulted. The hospital's doctors typically initiated conversations with local healers in cases where patients revealed that they had journeyed to and sought treatment in Hot Springs on an earlier occasion or when treatment needs exceeded the abilities of Army and Navy staff.[69] An example of the latter can be seen in the case of George Harrington, who came to the hospital on March 3, 1907, suffering from blurred vision in the right eye. Upon examination, doctors detected "copper colored scars" on the man's legs and "mucous patches" on his mouth and tongue. A syphilitic diagnosis followed shortly thereafter, and in addition to treating Harrington with mercury, the resident surgeon contacted Paul Vaughan, a surgical specialist with a large venereal clientele. Responding to the surgeon's request for help, Vaughan agreed to examine Harrington himself. After doing so, he sent the hospital a short letter explaining that Harrington had a "retinitis with slight inflammation of the optic papula." "Push his mercury to the limit," Vaughan advised (box 17).

Army and Navy doctors' reluctance to afford the Wassermann a place of diagnostic primacy may have stemmed from their interactions with Hot Springs' private practitioners.[70] While similarly employing it, many of the city's venereal specialists looked askance at this new serological procedure, arguing that "too much stress is being laid on the Wassermann and too little upon a carefully taken history and painstaking examination."[71] Though recognizing that "you cannot always depend on what [your patients] may tell you," throughout the early twentieth century the healers of Hot Springs stressed the need for a "detailed history" in all suspected venereal cases.[72] As one local doctor had it, "the Wassermann test is uncertain."[73]

With the passage of time, the views of the broader American medical community increasingly aligned with these sentiments. By the 1920s, the Wassermann's limitations were more apparent, prompting doctors to invest newfound levels of diagnostic importance in patient testimony.[74] More than likely, this not only provided doctors with a more accurate knowledge of syphilis but also improved their success in the treatment of this venereal disease.

This was certainly true for Andrew Magyar. A thirty-eight-year-old Hungarian native, Magyar entered Army and Navy on February 24, 1911, complaining of "rheumatic pains" in the chest and hips. Though presenting no physical evidence of a venereal infection, Magyar confessed to having been administered "local treatment" for a "hard chancre . . . about a year ago." This raised doctors' suspicions, and so they ordered a Wassermann test. When the results of this procedure came back positive, Magyar was put on a regimen of Salvarsan. Soon reported to be "very well," on April 26, 1911, a doctor noted that "this patient is leaving the hospital today" (box 34).[75]

Improved therapeutic outcomes like this were a product of the new medical environment created by the revoking of Army and Navy's venereal ban. While those who traveled to Hot Springs before 1910 displayed a great deal of reticence when asked about their venereal histories, patients admitted to the hospital after 1910 responded to these inquiries with candor, transparency, and frankness. Ultimately, the diagnostic insights provided through case histories facilitated doctors' growing venereological confidence to a much greater extent than did the Wassermann test.

Conclusion

As the second decade of the twentieth century began, a revolution in resident doctors' knowledge of syphilis was afoot. What had once been an amorphous, unstable disease entity was being transformed into a well-defined, stable one. At first glance, it may seem that this transformation owed largely to the introduction of the Wassermann test, which became a fixture of Army and Navy's venereological capabilities at the precise moment (1910) that doctors' difficulties in diagnosing syphilis became a thing of the past. However, as this analysis has shown, there was no "laboratory revolution" in early twentieth-century venereology. Instead, it was ultimately a rather old source of information that enabled hospital doctors to decipher syphilis's mysteries: the case history. With the repeal of a regulation refusing the admittance of venereal cases, hospital staff suddenly had access to a vast repository of data gathered through patient testimony, and the knowledge resulting from this proved key to their improved understanding of syphilis. At every step of the way, information acquired from personal interviews drove doctors' use of the Wassermann test, guiding their decisions about when to employ it, how to interpret it, and how to incorporate its results into the medical care provided to patients. Thus, for all its help, the Wassermann played a secondary role in the shifting perceptions of syphilis that emerged from Army and Navy after 1910. In the end, the new, modern disease construct that emerged from within the walls of this hospital was less the result of changes in global technology than of local policies and their impact on doctor-patient interactions.

Though syphilis's identity changed dramatically during these years, in Hot Springs, the source of its identity changed *not at all*. As in the late nineteenth century, throughout the early twentieth century local actors continued to exert a profound influence over the shape syphilis acquired within this southern city. It was those who mostly closely interacted with syphilis, and in particular, the city's largely unknown venereal patients, rather than elites in far-off places who determined how Hot Springs would think of and respond to this menace to the nation's private and public health. As the next chapter illustrates, these typically anonymous actors continued to influence America's battles with sexually transmitted diseases into the 1920s and 1930s.

CHAPTER FOUR

The Hot Springs VD Clinic, 1920–1937

In the winter of 1936, Minnie Lee Ishcomer left her home in Idabel, Oklahoma, and journeyed to Hot Springs, Arkansas. Thirty years old, white, poor, and the victim of a long-standing venereal infection, Ishcomer came to Hot Springs hoping to obtain treatment at the VD clinic operated there by the United States Public Health Service (PHS). Her experience was less than satisfactory. Because the clinic officially admitted only acute, infectious VD cases, Ishcomer was initially denied entrance—on the grounds that she was "not a danger to the public health." She passed her first few days in Hot Springs in search of food and shelter. Without money, she made her way to a bus station where a police officer found her "in a very serious condition." Taken back to the clinic, she received a few days' treatment. Soon after her release, a PHS official angrily wired the health officer in Ishcomer's home county that "such cases will not be treated in the future."[1]

The treatment Minnie Lee Ishcomer received likely did little to improve her health.[2] Nevertheless, her story sheds light on a relatively unexplored site of public health work in the early twentieth-century US South.[3] The opening of the Hot Springs VD clinic in 1921 followed on extensive antivenereal initiatives carried out by the US military during World War One. Marking the beginning of the civilian side of the federal government's campaign against syphilis and gonorrhea (which would continue with the Tuskegee Study of Untreated Syphilis in the Negro Male and the Chicago Syphilis Control Project), the clinic remained open into the 1940s. Throughout the interwar period, Hot Springs sat on the front lines of the PHS's war against VD, and although its efforts were largely unsuccessful, the clinic's history points toward a more complex understanding of this chapter in the early twentieth-century's "venereal peril."

First and foremost, the story of the Hot Springs clinic complicates the "science vs. sin" framework at the heart of much historical scholarship on VD. According to many accounts, the federal government's failure to adequately address syphilis and gonorrhea in the early twentieth century owed to the fact that PHS officials saw these diseases through a moral prism—one that relegated therapeutic approaches to "secondary" importance.[4] Had the state seen VD as "a public health problem rather than a moral problem," these studies suggest, its disease-control efforts would have been much more successful.[5] In Hot Springs, however, syphilis and gonorrhea persisted *in spite of* the federal government's adoption of a generally "broadminded and scientific" understanding of VD.[6] Privileging medicine over morality, during the 1920s and 1930s, clinic doctors administered over one million shots of Salvarsan and mercury to more than sixty thousand patients—black as well as white, male as well as female. The key problem was not morality but *poverty*. Though recognizing that the country's problems with VD were ultimately traceable to "faults in our economic structure," the PHS proved unable to solve the root problem of poverty—its adoption of a secular mindset notwithstanding.[7]

In addition to illustrating that the early twentieth-century struggle against syphilis was both ideological *and* material, this chapter also points to the central role local, nonstate actors played in shaping the federal government's response to this disease. Just as Minnie Lee Ischomer upended PHS policies, over the course of the 1920s and 1930s, both visiting patients and local inhabitants exerted a notable influence on the work of the Hot Springs clinic, transforming a site originally dedicated to scientific research and traditional antivenereal measures (mass testing and treating, the incarceration of prostitutes, etc.) into something centered on the pursuit of extramedical, economically based solutions to the country's venereal woes. While one of the long-standing themes in VD historiography is the abusive power often wielded by state and federal governments, within Hot Springs, there were countervailing forces at play—including those that frustrated federal aims, empowered the sick, and created new opportunities for health and well-being.

These opportunities, however, did not apply equally to all of the clinic's patients. Though many of its initiatives benefited patients regardless of race or sex, the PHS often extended special privileges to white health seekers. Some of these preferential arrangements were informal, while others—Camp Garraday, for instance, a transient facility on the outskirts of Hot Springs that provided food, shelter, work opportunities, and domiciliary care to the clinic's white male patients—were institutional. For African American men and women, by contrast, the Hot Springs experience was often marked by hostility and discrimination. All of this demonstrates the cultural currents coursing through the PHS facility, whose director—Oliver C. Wenger—declared syphilis and gonorrhea important "from the standpoint of race conservation."[8] Offering insights into the racial and gendered aspects of the federal government's campaign against syphilis and gonorrhea, the story of the Hot Springs VD clinic adds to recent analyses of the Tuskegee study demonstrating how forcefully eugenics pervaded the PHS's early twentieth-century disease-control efforts.[9]

Creating the Clinic

The "venereal peril" reached its apex during the First World War. Armed with scientific methods of diagnosis, doctors found that a surprisingly high number of prospective US military recruits suffered from VD. Hoping to head off a manpower shortage, in 1917 Congress created the Committee on Training Camp Activities—an organization that sought to curb the venereal scourge through the forced incarceration of prostitutes, the provision of medical services for infected soldiers, and the establishment of "wholesome" alternatives to the vice-ridden recreational opportunities commonly found in cantonment zones.[10] The following year Congress passed the Chamberlain-Kahn Act, which created the PHS's Division of Venereal Diseases, and allocated two million dollars for the establishment of free VD clinics across the country.[11] As the war came to a close, Washington followed up on these efforts by conducting a nationwide VD survey.

Each of these developments drew attention to Hot Springs. Throughout the war, military authorities fretted over Little Rock's Camp Pike, a training facility whose VD rates were reportedly "the [highest] by far of any camp or cantonment in the United States."[12] According to local commanders, Camp Pike's reputation as a hotbed of sexual sickness owed to its proximity to Hot Springs, where prostitution had been legal since the late nineteenth century and where brothels enjoyed a reputation as home to the profession's "aristocrats."[13] In August 1918, Camp Pike's commanders ordered the closure of Hot Springs' numerous "houses of immorality."[14] Municipal authorities reluctantly complied, but the federal government's interest in Hot Springs did not end. While conducting their postwar VD survey, government officials grew increasingly anxious about the city's "serious medical and social problems," observing that Hot Springs was home to an increasing population of venereally afflicted "indigents" and an entirely "inadequate" public health infrastructure.[15]

From the federal perspective, syphilitic health seekers represented an "interstate menace."[16] The PHS was determined to "protect the rest of the country" from those who traversed it with a venereal infection.[17] Opening a clinic in Hot Springs devoted to rendering the afflicted noninfectious seemed the best means of accomplishing this goal. Because patients traveled here from all parts of the country, constituted a diverse racial and socioeconomic makeup, and encompassed the full range of syphilitic infections, the PHS also found in Hot Springs an unprecedented opportunity for research. Indeed, given its desire to create "new and better methods to fight venereal diseases," the federal government looked to Hot Springs as a place that would "be of great help to the State boards of health . . . in carrying on their campaign to prevent the spread of venereal infection."[18] Finally, establishing a long-term presence here would also allow the government to continue its wartime campaign against "houses of immorality," while transforming a parochial medical culture.[19]

In late 1920 the PHS drew up plans for the facility, obtained $300,000 in construction funds and selected Oliver C. Wenger, one of the country's leading venereologists, as director.[20] Born in St. Louis in 1884, Wenger obtained his MD from St. Louis University in 1908. During the First World War, he served in the Medical Corps of the Missouri National Guard, later traveling to England and France as part of a sanitary squad involved in VD control.[21] His time in Europe convinced Wenger to devote all his efforts to venereology. According to a contemporary, Wenger's idea of heaven was a place containing "unlimited syphilis," and of course, "unlimited facilities to treat it."[22] In 1919, Wenger joined the PHS Division of Venereal Disease. Before becoming director at Hot Springs, his first assignment was the national VD survey.

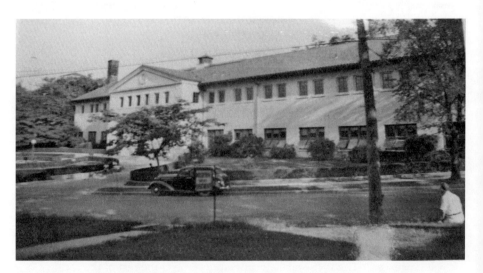

This 1921 photograph shows the entrance to the Hot Springs VD clinic, a two-story building with separate floors for bathing and treatment. Courtesy of University of Arkansas for Medical Sciences Historical Research Center

Inside the Clinic

With an inaugural budget of $40,000, the clinic opened in August 1921.[23] In its first year, five hundred patients received treatment; by 1936, 61,930 patients had wound their way through and a total of 1.2 million injections of mercury and Salvarsan had been administered. Who were these individuals? How did their circumstances, needs, and experiences differ? How did prevailing ideas about VD influence Hot Springs' response to syphilis? And how did the clinic's campaign develop over the course of the 1920s and 1930s?

On one level, the PHS's day-to-day work reflected the widespread belief that VD constituted the "wages of sin"—a sign of sexual immorality. In lectures given by clinic personnel, patients learned that their illnesses were the result of "ignorance and [their] own misconduct." This message of personal irresponsibility also found its way into the clinic's official instructions, which warned patients not to "loaf downtown" between treatments. Above all other commandments stood one: "DON'T GET INTO TROUBLE."[24] Contending that one's success in combating syphilis or gonorrhea was simply a matter of "choice," Wenger counseled his patients that they had the power to "decide which road" they would "travel."[25]

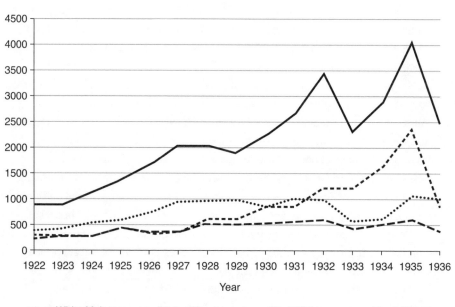

VD Cases Admitted to the Hot Springs Clinic, 1922–1936

In keeping with these views about self-responsibility, Wenger's early strategies for combating syphilis revolved primarily around the uncovering and treatment of infectious venereal cases. In order to achieve the first of these goals, the Hot Springs VD clinic employed a social worker whose job it was to investigate the "social relations and home conditions" of each patient. Endeavoring to determine the source of a particular syphilitic's infection and to gather information regarding "other persons likely to have been exposed" to said infection, the social worker participated in one of the central facets of the successful antivenereal program: case tracking.[26] In these efforts Wenger was assiduous, for between the 1920s and 1930s the head of the city's government-run medical facility regularly dispatched letters to local health officers all across the country, letters in which the PHS agent asked that the identified sources of his patients' illnesses be contacted, tested, and if necessary treated until rendered noninfectious.

Typical was the case of James Daugherty, a thirty-seven-year-old white male who upon entering Wenger's clinic identified a woman named Beatrice Brown (of Monticello, Arkansas) as the source of his sickness. Obtaining this woman's full address, Wenger informed the Arkansas State Board of Health of Brown's whereabouts, asking that a copy of the local officer's investigative report be forwarded to his clinic.[27] As part of his agency's case-tracking efforts, Wenger at times pledged his personal "cooperation" in these matters, offering to treat those identified as sources of infection at the Hot Springs VD clinic.[28] And in some instances, those listed as possible sources of exposure did make their way to Wenger's facility, as was the case with Vida Ward, a woman named by a thirty-one-year-old syphilitic from Brookston, Texas, as a likely source of infection.[29]

Upon entering Hot Springs, patients like Ward were "expected to make arrangements to pay [their] own room and board."[30] Given that the minimum course of therapy lasted between twenty and thirty weeks, the PHS recommended that "no patient should go to Hot Springs without at least a return ticket and $100 in cash." Such expectations often clashed with reality. Wenger observed that "less than five percent of these indigent persons had funds with which to maintain themselves while receiving free treatment."[31] Many arrived "without one cent of money."[32] In 1931 the average applicant carried not "$100 in cash" but $15.43. The following year, this average fell to $8.76.[33] A "dumping ground of many indigents" during the 1920s and 1930s, Hot Springs became the preserve of all sorts of "unfortunate people" who "slept out on the hillside or in alleys, begging food from door to door . . . or looking for food in garbage cans."[34] As Wenger admitted, "the great majority left . . . before they could receive enough treatment to give them any real benefit."[35]

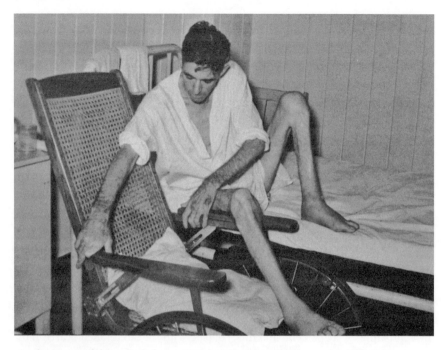

As the image of this crippled, emaciated male patient indicates, the difficulties confronting those who traveled to the Hot Springs VD clinic included not only venereal infection but also poverty, hunger, and general disability. Courtesy of University of Arkansas for Medical Sciences Historical Research Center

One of this "great majority" was Virgil Oren Adams. A native of Clovis, New Mexico, during the early 1930s Adams made several visits to the Hot Springs VD clinic. Each time, he "ran out of funds" after only a few weeks and being "sick and weak from lack of food and sleep" was forced to leave. In 1934 he wrote to President Roosevelt seeking assistance for yet another clinic trip. "I have been fighting syphilis since 1927," Adams wrote, adding that he was "very much interested in . . . getting rid of this terrible disease." Declaring that he was "absolutely broke," Adams begged Roosevelt for a letter to take "as a recommendation for treatments at Hot Springs." "Anything you can do in my behalf," he pleaded, would be "highly appreciated."[36]

Cases like Adams's were a "daily occurrence."[37] While poverty hampered patients' chances of recovery, so did the advanced state of their ailments. Most venereal sufferers came to Hot Springs long after contracting syphilis or gonorrhea. Most had not received more than a few shots of mercury or Salvarsan, and many relied only on cheap, ineffective patent medicines.[38] Their illnesses were chronic and generally immune to existing remedies. With disease burrowed deep in their bodies, few had any hope of ever being free from VD.

Realities such as these inspired a modicum of sympathy among clinic doctors. Particularly worrying to Wenger was the fate of ex-servicemen. Disappointed by the fact that during World War I, "our young American manhood" was often "unable to serve because of venereal diseases," Wenger observed hundreds of infected former soldiers seeking admittance to the Hot Springs clinic during the early 1920s. Like most patients, they were "nomads, seeking treatment here and there." Particularly troubling was the fact that these veterans were beginning to form families and had entered "the best years [of their lives] from an economic standpoint." All of them needed medical attention; none were in a position to pay. Such matters made the treatment and control of syphilis and gonorrhea a national priority, he urged, especially "from the standpoint of race conservation."[39]

Language such as this dovetailed with contemporary eugenic discourse. Like other eugenicists, Wenger's interest in "race conservation" stemmed from anxieties over white racial purity and integrity. Over the course of the nineteenth and early twentieth centuries, birth rates among native-born white women declined by approximately 45 percent, and this, coupled with the simultaneous arrival of millions of "new immigrants" from southern and eastern Europe, prompted fears of "race suicide" among the nation's political and cultural elite.[40] Speaking to these fears, New York City gynecologist Abraham Wolbarst opined that "the flower of our land, the mothers of our future citizenship, are being mutilated and unsexed by surgical life-saving diseases, particularly gonorrhea."[41] Sentiments such as Wolbarst's were widely held by PHS officials, including Oliver Wenger—whose eugenic beliefs scholars have also found evidence of in his later work in Tuskegee and Chicago.[42]

In response to the financial obstacles that prevented so many patients from remaining in Hot Springs for between twenty and thirty weeks, the PHS sought means of accelerating the therapeutic process. Among the myriad venereological experiments conducted at Hot Springs, none loomed larger than those undertaken in the Salvarsan room. During the early 1920s clinic personnel began "the intensive and continuous plan of treatment."[43] In the typical VD clinic, patients received one dose of Salvarsan per week; in Hot Springs, they would receive twice that amount.[44]

Derived largely from arsenic, a highly toxic substance, Salvarsan was a frightening remedy. While more effective than mercury, its use was accompanied by a panoply of side effects—from the mild (dermatitis, gastrointestinal distress) to the severe (ocular damage, cardiac distress, edema). In rare cases, death resulted.

In a review of 6,308 syphilis patients admitted between 1922 and 1932, Wenger counted a total of 225 adverse reactions to Salvarsan—including three fatalities from arsenical poisoning.[45] It appears that severe reactions to Salvarsan were more common here than elsewhere.[46] Cognizant of the fact that "the duration of anti-syphilitic treatment at the Hot Springs clinic is for a relatively short time," Wenger's staff rushed to experiment with untested modes of therapy. The adoption of an "intensive and continuous plan of treatment" contributed to the clinic's high rate of serious complications.[47]

Such was certainly the case for Forrest LaPrade. A twenty-four-year-old Texan who arrived in Hot Springs in March 1930, LaPrade's original intention was to "boil out nicotine and malaria" through the city's "healing waters." Directed to Wenger's clinic for a physical, LaPrade was found to be syphilitic. Over the next few weeks he received seven shots of Salvarsan and eleven of mercury. His condition then worsened.[48]

On May 2, 1930, LaPrade complained of a "slight oedma" of the face, which his physician noted was "characteristic of arsenical poisoning." By the next day, he displayed a "face intensely swollen," along with a fever and an accelerated heart rate. After being diagnosed with erysipelas, LaPrade was transferred by a friend to a nearby hospital, where for twenty-eight days he experienced "untold agonies." Hoping to heal his swollen face, from which dripped "large drops of yellow corruption," LaPrade's doctors covered him with a white, glue-like paste, a remedy that produced a constant itching sensation that left the Texan "at the point of death." "I was actually skinned alive," LaPrade later said, describing how the itching left him "scaled like a fish." Unable to sleep, LaPrade's condition was so bad that his body "trembled like a leaf and even shook or quivered the bed." "I suffered, cried, and prayed as one who was in the doorway of Hell," he recalled with horror. "But for the Lord, I would have been six feet of earth."[49]

Although few patients faced an ordeal like Forrest LaPrade's, the clinic's other experiments also encountered serious difficulties. Perhaps the most significant obstacle was patients' inability to remain in Hot Springs for sufficient periods of time. A case in point is an experiment conducted in the early 1930s involving a procedure known as surgical diathermy. Performed on a group of 288 female patients suffering from gonorrhea-induced chronic endocervicitis, the experiment entailed the use of a "high-frequency current," which clinic doctors applied to the women's cervical canals. Though designed as a two-month study, seventeen subjects vanished after one week, and ninety-eight more left the city between the second and seventh weeks. While the 173 subjects still present at the two-month point stated that their vaginal discharges had been "greatly lessened" and that they were "extremely pleased with the results," on the whole, the study's findings were marred by a high rate of attrition.[50]

Difficulties such as these hindered the clinic's efforts to produce "new and better methods to fight venereal diseases."[51] A report from the PHS's Division of Venereal Diseases spoke in disappointed terms: "It was hoped that this clinic would prove useful from a research standpoint, but because of the transient character of the patients, results thus far have not been up to expectations."[52] So caught off guard was the PHS by these unanticipated realities that even seemingly simple, straightforward tasks such as record keeping proved well-nigh impossible. As early as 1923, federal officials had begun drawing attention to the "very incomplete" nature of the facility's case files; as one observer put it, "Records are not kept by the clinic in such form as to enable figures to be shown indicating the number being examined each day."[53] And as late as 1936, clinic personnel were still reporting on the "comparatively small number of treatments" given to patients—a reference to how few individuals completed a full course of antivenereal treatment.[54]

If patients' financial misery hindered the clinic's hopes of being "useful from a research standpoint," so too did their *physical* circumstances. Because the overwhelming majority of the city's patients exhibited the secondary and tertiary manifestations of syphilis, much of the research undertaken here dealt not with methods for preventing the spread of VD but instead with developing cures for those with noncommunicable infections. In reorienting medical research around therapies and procedures that were both dangerous and of limited applicability, patients undercut the clinic's original mission.

Wenger's experiments with a device known as the Kettering hypetherm provide evidence of how the clinic's brief was undermined by patients' physical situation. In May 1936, Wenger received word of a "special cabinet" that the Mayo clinic had begun testing on some of its gonorrhea patients. Although noting that it was "still in the experimental stage," Wenger was so favorably impressed by the preliminary results that he urged his superiors to acquire one of these pyrexic machines and send it to Hot Springs for "experimental purposes." "Imagine curing early gonorrhea by five or six heat treatments, in three weeks time," he wired Washington.[55] Shortly after this, Wenger got his wish, and after arriving in late 1936, the Kettering hypetherm remained in "almost daily use" for the next two years.[56] Yet despite the initial optimism, the clinic's studies of gonorrheal "heat treatment" failed to yield much in the way of more effective disease-control methods.

Why was this? Chiefly, because the cabinet's applicability was limited to an incredibly select group of patients—those with the "most severe and incapacitat-

ing complications" derived from gonorrhea. Based on the finding that gonococci raised in vitro were incapable of withstanding temperatures above 105.8 degrees Fahrenheit, the hypetherm was found to produce extraordinary results in
cases of gonorrheal arthritis and gonorrheal ophthalmia. However, the device was
"not without its dangers": typical complications included a "persistently fast
pulse," "slow and irregular breathing," "derangement of the heat center," delir-
ium, convulsions, and coma. In many cases, patients had to be temporarily removed from the cabinet, and at times, "permanent discontinuance of treatment" was required. One particularly unsettling outcome involved a man whose
temperature rose to 109.2 degrees Fahrenheit; "fortunately," a study on the new
therapeutic device observed, "death did not result." On account of these "many
and varied" negative side effects, clinic personnel ruled out the Kettering's use
in minor forms of gonorrheal disease—including epididymitis and prostatitis—
and concluded that the device was only indicated among gonorrhea patients
who were "totally disabled from gainful occupation."[57] While many of Hot
Springs' gonorrhea patients may have experienced serious complications, nation-
ally, patients did not.

Healing the "Other": Women and African Americans at the Hot Springs VD Clinic

Because their attempts to accelerate the curative process largely failed, Wenger's
staff also investigated ways of keeping patients within Hot Springs for longer periods of time. This search for extramedical means of disease control had a racial
foundation, one that becomes clear through an examination of doctors' experiences with female patients. Initially, Wenger and his staff harbored quite negative attitudes toward women, who were seen as "uncontrolled spreaders of infection" and a "menace to the community at large."[58] With the passage of time,
however, clinic personnel became increasingly sympathetic to the plight of female health seekers—even those who supported themselves through prostitution while receiving treatment. From these sentiments (which extended only to
whites) emerged a nontraditional disease-control program, one rooted not only
in testing and treatment but also in socioeconomic measures—including financial aid for food and housing.

Wenger's first few years in Hot Springs were characterized by an intensive
crackdown on the city's red-light districts, which had reopened in the aftermath
of World War One. Hoping to prevent local brothels from recovering their former
strength, in January 1921 the PHS presented an ultimatum to municipal authorities, explaining that unless the city abolished its regulated district, the agency

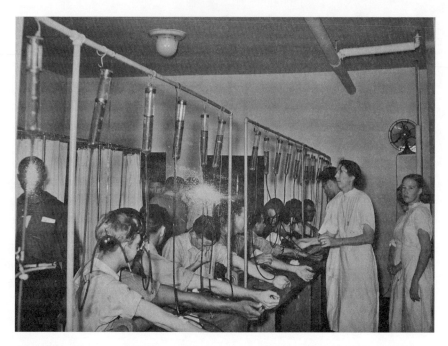

Throughout the 1920s and 1930s, clinic personnel treated syphilis with Salvarsan via the "intensive and continuous plan." Engineered for mass administration, the Salvarsan room had the capacity to treat fifty patients simultaneously. For an especially impassioned description of this clinical apparatus, see Paul de Kruif, *The Sweeping Wind: A Memoir* (New York: Harcourt, Brace, and World, 1962), 206–7. Courtesy of University of Arkansas for Medical Sciences Historical Research Center

would quarantine all individuals who came to Hot Springs seeking treatment for disease—venereal or otherwise. Recognizing that it would "prove a great financial blow to the city if this patronage were lost," the PHS argued that it was "absolutely inconsistent to permit men to go there for the cure and, at the same time be exposed to reinfection through the agency of an open red-light district." Women too would be subject to these measures, as some of the female patients in Hot Springs were prostitutes who "carry on their profession while under treatment."[59]

That women would be included was made clear by a report Wenger received from the Interdepartmental Social Hygiene Department in 1922. A governmental entity tasked with investigating the relationship between prostitution and VD, the department in 1921 sent an agent named Blanche Young to Hot Springs. Upon questioning a few girls "of the prostitute type" found within the city's public dance halls, she concluded that no progress against VD would be forthcoming unless the federal government abolished its system of regulated prostitution. One of the prostitutes Young met with informed her that "she had gone to the city for medical treatment and was under the care of a private physician." On another occasion, Young encountered a "very fast looking girl enter[ing] an automobile occupied by three young men who were obviously under the influence of liquor." "A little later," Young continued, "I saw this automobile stop and the men 'pick up' two girls. This was about 11:43 PM. The men talked to the girls on the street, inducing them to enter the car, immediately driving off. The next day I recognized in both the G.U. [genitourinary] and syphilis clinics one of the girls who was present in the dance hall."[60]

Reports such as these inclined Wenger toward an all-out assault on the city's red-light district. As during wartime, Hot Springs' response to this federal ultimatum was regretful compliance. The death of the city's physician-mayor J. W. McClendon—"the leader of the wide-open town policy"—eased Washington's task. With the removal of this "obstacle," the PHS convinced local law enforcement officials to fall in line.[61] By the summer of 1922, five brothels had been shut down; by 1923, their number had been reduced by half.[62] These results bore out the federal government's conclusion that local personnel had been "very successful" in "eliminating houses of prostitution" in Hot Springs.[63]

This assessment proved premature, however. The interwar years brought new life to prostitution. While initially complying with the PHS, steep declines in revenue from saloons and bawdy houses prompted municipal officials to change their minds.[64] In the late 1920s the city's mayor "[threw] the town wide open" to prostitution, and in the next decade, cases of "female patients street-walking or soliciting" were "almost of daily occurrence."[65] The clinic did little to oppose this challenge to federal authority. A 1934 visitor to the city remarked that Hot Springs was "the only national park where gambling, imbibing, and prostitution go unmolested."[66]

What explains this reversal? For one, it appears that clinic personnel had little appetite for prolonged conflict with the array of local forces (officials, doctors, and brothel owners) opposed to the abolition of prostitution. Since the late nineteenth century, local prostitutes had been allowed to conduct their business without police interference, provided brothel owners and their "inmates" paid a monthly "fine" that fed into city coffers. Such a system had the full support of Hot Springs' private medical practitioners, who regarded organized prostitution as one of those "necessary evils" that had existed "from time immemorial" and that therefore required regulation and control rather than abolition.[67] While local healers had rather discriminatory and prejudiced racial views, they took a notably sympathetic

and enlightened view toward sex workers: as one of their number put it, "Prostitutes themselves need protection and have claims on the humanity of the law."[68]
Of course, their acceptance of the practice likely stemmed at least in part from
the fact that prostitutes constituted an important source of income for resort doctors. Regardless, it is clear that by the early twentieth century, prostitution was
an entrenched and incredibly profitable part of the city's medical, legal, and social environment, and the trade's practitioners—said to be "on the courtesan
order"—were are a far cry from the impoverished and desperate women who
daily sold their bodies in many other parts of the country. "It would not do to call
them prostitutes," Archie Cowles observed in a December 10, 1905, letter, "for
they are aristocrats in their profession."

Also important in understanding this reversal are the interactions clinic personnel had with female patients—many of whom sold their bodies for sex while
seeking VD treatment. Consider the experience of a "young white woman" from
Tennessee named "OJ." Orphaned since childhood, OJ had grown up at the
House of the Good Shepherd in Memphis. With "limited" opportunities, she
then supported herself largely through prostitution—by which she contracted
both syphilis and gonorrhea. Upon arriving in Hot Springs, OJ found work as a
boardinghouse maid. Subsequently accused by her landlady of "running around
with men," OJ found herself back on the streets. For the remainder of her stay,
she supported herself through prostitution, a decision she defended with three
words: "I must eat." While concerned over the number of "boy friends" this "more
than ordinarily attractive" woman had infected, Wenger sympathized with OJ's
plight, explaining to his superiors that "she was a good patient and reported regularly for treatment." Summarizing her case, the PHS agent conceded that "it is
hard to be chaste and hungry."[69]

Interactions with patients like OJ had a dramatic impact on clinicians, who
came to accept prostitution not as an indication of immorality but as a consequence of the adverse circumstances many female patients faced.[70] In one of his
earliest reports, Wenger spoke of the "large number of female patients" who arrived in Hot Springs with "no funds" and "no friends." With work "scarce" in
the city, many of these women—in a "much discouraged" state—were "forced by
dire necessity to support [themselves] by prostitution."[71] The experiences of patients like OJ were "not unique nor unusual, but exactly what goes on as these
transients move across the country in their efforts to receive free medical service."[72] Criticizing those who argued that prostitution could not be tolerated,
Wenger explained that "as social workers and health officers, we must change our

own attitude and remember that we ourselves would become transients seeking medical services if they were not available at home. This is only natural."[73]

Consistent with his new understanding of prostitution, Wenger's interactions with female patients displayed a lack of moralizing. Fully aware of the fact that "the whole subject of prophylaxis is T.N.T." (that is, trinitrotoluene, a highly explosive chemical compound) and that public discussions of contraception "might innocently start some unwelcome comment," Wenger nevertheless presented lectures on how to "prevent a second infection," endorsing the use of condoms (which he held to be "fairly safe . . . providing [they do] not break") and teaching women "the value of prophylaxis and also contraceptives, or birth control methods."[74] A typical lesson began with a discussion of female anatomy and concluded with demonstrations of birth control techniques. While initially concerned about how female patients would react to these frank methods, Wenger reported that "there has been no embarrassment on the part of the volunteer subjects or the patients looking on. The remarks and questions asked during the demonstrations are amazing."[75]

The clinic's female patients also encouraged Wenger to search for economic solutions to the country's VD epidemic. Consider the 1933 case of "Mrs. W." A white, college-educated woman who "came here all the way from old Mexico" after having been deserted by her husband (who infected her with syphilis) and having "suffered losses in the general depression," upon arriving in Hot Springs, Mrs. W. at first lived "in the colored section of town with a colored woman." When this woman's relatives moved in, Mrs. W. informed clinic personnel that she was "planning to 'hitchhike' her way back to Nogales, Arizona," where friends would take her home. Believing such a trip would be "practically impossible," Wenger turned to local welfare agencies, "who agreed to pay half of her fare." The remainder was "made up by clinic personnel."[76]

What prompted Wenger's generosity in this case, it seems, was the fact that Mrs. W had been made to depend on the "bounty of a colored maid." "Imagine a cultured woman in this predicament," he said of Mrs. W, informing his superiors that if only maintenance could have been arranged "for a longer period of time," she would have again become "self-supporting."[77] Wenger was clearly troubled by the specter of a world in which middle- and upper-class whites suddenly found themselves lowered beneath the socioeconomic level of the country's African American inhabitants; his intervention here speaks to the role racial beliefs played in his evolving views on syphilis. In keeping with this, it bears noting that Wenger's annual reports never made mention of black men or women whose difficulties elicited the kinds of financial support provided for "cultured" patients like Mrs. W.

Like OJ and Mrs. W., most of the women who made their way to the Hot Springs clinic in the 1930s were white. During the clinic's formative years, white women never accounted for more than one-fifth of the clinic's annual caseload. Between 1928 and 1936, however, their numbers steadily grew, reaching a peak of 2,353 in 1935—a year in which they represented nearly one-third of all patients treated. During the same time period, African Americans' share of the clinic's annual caseload declined from 36.9 percent to 20.3 percent—a trend especially evident among women.[78] Those who managed to make their way to Hot Springs experienced exceptional financial difficulties. Between 1922 and 1932, for example, the number of African American visitors listed in the "unskilled labor" category was "nearly twice as high" as the comparable figure for whites.[79] Those still able to finance a stay here came to Hot Springs later in the course of their infections than did whites, and in addition to presenting less curable forms of illness, they also left Wenger's clinic much earlier than did white men and women. As late as 1940, a study revealed that whereas the average white syphilitic received twelve shots of Salvarsan, blacks received only nine.[80]

Within the clinic, black patients received a less sympathetic response than did white health seekers such as Mrs. W. or OJ. For example, shortly after entering the clinic on September 3, 1927, Charley Wade Bradshaw—a twenty-five-year-old black man employed as a porter by the Oklahoma City Railway Power House— was diagnosed with neurosyphilis and placed on a regimen of mercury. For six weeks, Bradshaw's savings enabled him to rent a room at a colored hotel, but on October 19, he was reported "AWOL." One year later, an Oklahoma City law firm supplied the reason for this abrupt departure. Coming to Hot Springs after company doctors "advised him that he had bad blood," Bradshaw left after running out of money for room and board. As an attorney informed Wenger, Bradshaw was "in a bad condition physically," and because he had "no means whatever," anyone who tried to help him "will have to do so at their expense."[81]

Wenger apparently made no effort to pay for Bradshaw's expenses, despite his recognition of the socioeconomic inequalities that imperiled black health.[82] While concurring that venereal diseases were "playing havoc within the Negro population of the country," he criticized those who interpreted these findings as evidence of African Americans' "absolute lack of morality." The observed differential between whites and blacks, commented Wenger, "does not mean that there is a considerable difference in the morals of these different groups." The critical variable was African Americans' "social economic status"—in particular, their "more limited" educational and employment opportunities. "When the social and economic backgrounds of the two races are considered," he concluded, "there seems to be little difference in the incidence of infection."[83]

But improving black health seekers' access to treatment required more than simply a rejection of the "syphilis-soaked negro" stereotype. When it came to removing institutional and economic barriers confronting African American VD patients, Wenger did little. He refused to challenge Hot Springs' adherence to Jim Crow, which confined African Americans to an "exterior observation" of all but two of the city's bathhouses. In addition to the "great disadvantage" they faced due to the "lack of proper accommodations in hotels and bathhouses," black patrons had fewer opportunities for securing therapeutic services than did whites. The Depression felled the one institution—the Woodmen of the Union Hospital—specifically catering to blacks.[84] Defending this inaction, Wenger wrote to his superiors in Washington that in matters that had the potential to court controversy, it was best to "let the State V.D. men do as they please."[85]

Racist attitudes were at times on display within the Hot Springs VD clinic. George Smith was a black man admitted in July 1925 after local authorities arrested him for "night prowling." While a judge ordered his release on the condition that he leave town, a Wassermann test revealed that Smith was infected with syphilis. Shortly after Wenger prevailed upon the city to permit his entrance into the PHS facility, trouble began. One day while receiving an injection of mercury, Smith reportedly became "impudent," and the doctor treating him "lost his temper and threatened to ruin" the man. Upon hearing of the incident, Wenger informed Smith to "remain away" from the clinic until the physician in question—a Dr. Abington—left. Though not expelling him, Wenger warned the doctor not to "cuss" the patients, and in his review of the case, the PHS official observed that Abington "was born and raised in the South, and [was] prejudiced toward all aggressive negroes."[86]

This was not the only reported instance of racial discrimination within the clinic. Another involved a black man discharged from the PHS facility after doctors alleged that he had been seen "peeping into the window of the female gynecologic douche room."[87] Later, in 1941, a PHS officer reportedly entered a number of "reputable Negro business places" in nearby Texarkana, arresting several "young ladies," and then transporting them to Hot Springs for treatment—all without testing them for venereal disease.[88] Though it is unclear how common such "Hitler-like" tactics were, their mere existence likely discouraged many black syphilitics from journeying to Hot Springs.[89]

Clinic to Camp

With female patients "forced by dire necessity" to turn to prostitution, blacks and whites alike facing "limited" employment opportunities, ex-servicemen becoming "nomads," and scores of patients "begging food from door to door," Wenger increasingly pivoted toward an environmental response to VD—one that addressed the disease's economic underpinnings. Also important here in forcing the PHS's hand was the community of Hot Springs itself, which became increasingly intolerant of the multitude of VD patients found "on the streets, begging, borrowing, and stealing." Local residents resoundingly objected to "the presence of such large numbers of indigent VD cases on the city streets."[90] On account of the pressure exerted by these outside forces, in the mid-1920s Wenger floated a request for funding to his superiors in Washington. The plan called for "some means of housing these indigent patients, or at least of providing them with sufficient food while they are under our care."[91] Unfortunately for the clinic's director, the 1920s was a decade of greatly reduced appetites for social spending. With the PHS facing a series of budget cuts, Wenger's calls for an extramedical answer to the clinic's dilemma fell on deaf ears.

With the onset of the Great Depression in 1929, however, life for the city's venereal health seekers changed markedly. Laying bare the relationship between socioeconomic status and health status, the unparalleled financial turmoil of the 1930s brought about not only mass unemployment and the loss of homes, farms, and bank accounts but also rising rates of malaria, typhoid, venereal disease, tuberculosis, hookworm, and pellagra. Particularly vulnerable to these preventable illnesses were the thousands upon thousands of men, women, and children separated from their families and hometowns; studies conducted by municipal authorities throughout the decade revealed the exceptional levels of medical hardship faced by communities with high numbers of migrants.[92] Often ineligible for local, county, or state-level assistance, migrants typically lacked any means whatsoever of obtaining medical services. Their plight was one of several health-related problems examined by the Committee on the Costs of Medical Care, a group of economists, physicians, and public health experts whose landmark 1932 study *Medical Care for the American People* argued that consumer-driven health care had failed to address the medical needs of the vast majority of the nation's population.[93]

The committee's message found a welcome reception within Washington. Throughout the 1930s, members of President Roosevelt's administration sought to create a "New Deal for Health," believing that increased public expenditures

could drive down morbidity and mortality rates and thus help create a more stable economic foundation for the future.[94] Within the PHS, syphilis and gonorrhea became prime candidates for intervention, as Thomas Parran and others
within the agency's VD division declared that the costs of leaving these diseases
untreated constituted an undue financial burden for businesses and taxpayers
alike. Deliberately distancing themselves from the idea that VD was the result of
sexual immorality, federal officials instead positioned this as the unwelcome by-
product of unregulated capitalism—as the symptom of an "unbalanced economic system."[95] Thus reframed as an environmental matter rather than an
individual one, syphilis control became part of the broader New Deal goal of
promoting national recovery via increased economic security.

Such views squared with Oliver Wenger's own beliefs. Repeatedly bearing witness to the travails of patients too poor to afford a course of treatment within
Hot Springs, during the 1930s, Wenger regularly railed against "the almost prohibitive cost of modern medical care."[96] The country's VD epidemic, he believed,
was largely "the product of faults in our economic structure," which compelled
sufferers to adopt a life of enforced transience and journey across the country to
"seek elsewhere the remedies they cannot obtain at home."[97] While in the past,
migratory behavior such as this posed little risk to public health, this was no longer the case: "as our *so-called civilization* advanced," he wrote in a 1936 essay,
communicable diseases steadily spread throughout the world, leading to the
modern-day situation in which there were "no frontiers for such diseases as
tuberculosis, gonorrhea, and syphilis."[98]

The federal government's response to the health crisis of the Great Depression
began in 1933, when the Federal Emergency Relief Administration issued a rul-
ing making funds available for the purchasing of medical care. Initially, administration aid was distributed so as to help individual families with unpaid doctors'
bills, but after two years, this rather personalized approach was augmented by a
cooperative insurance scheme overseen by the Resettlement Administration and
(after 1937) the Farm Security Administration. Run on the basis of a group pre-
payment system, this program significantly reduced the costs of medical care for
low-income Americans—particularly in the South, a region with fewer doctors,
fewer hospitals, and higher rates of morbidity and mortality than the rest of the
country.[99]

While beneficial, these programs did little to address migrants' medical needs.
As such, in 1938, the Farm Security Administration embarked on an even bolder
initiative, the cornerstone of which was a series of transient health centers. Constructed all across the country, these camps not only provided migrants with

food, water, and shelter but also offered a range of clinical services—including drug-based therapies, surgery, immunizations, pre- and postnatal care, dental care, and instruction in personal hygiene and nutrition. By the early 1940s, an estimated three hundred thousand Americans were enrolled in one of the government's migrant health plans.[100]

Hot Springs played a central role in the government's response to the health crisis of the 1930s. During the Depression, when the city was "swamped with applicants seeking medical aid," local authorities complained about an increase in "begging, borrowing, and stealing."[101] Many of these applicants, wrote Wagner, belonged to a "much higher type group," individuals who in normal times would not have had to avail themselves of free, government-provided services.[102] Aware of the ways his clinic was "causing objection and criticism from certain groups of citizens," in 1933 Wenger again asked for federal housing for indigent patients. His next budget included monies courtesy of the Arkansas Transient Bureau (ATB), a branch of the Federal Transient Bureau, to provide "free room and board" at "$1.00 per day per patient," as well as funds for hospitalization, telegrams, minor emergencies, and transportation home.[103]

During its first month in operation, the ATB provided shelter, clothing, food, and medical attention to over twenty-three hundred VD patients—black as well as white, female as well as male. The program reaped immediate dividends: according to state officials, only one year after the implementation of Wenger's "maintenance" plans, the number of venereal health seekers leaving Hot Springs noninfectious increased by 38 percent.[104] In January 1934, Wenger wired Washington to praise the ATB for "giving out free room and board," likewise noting that as a result of this "most of the old patients are remaining because they are getting free room and board and are taking more treatment."[105]

While generally true, statements such as these masked the racially divergent impacts of the transient program. Though the ATB provided maintenance funds for both black and white patients, the clinic's data indicates that the proportion of African American patients housed in local hotels and boarding houses was 9 percent lower than the comparable rate for whites. Such a disparity reflected two unfortunate realities: the city's adherence to Jim Crow, which drastically restricted the number of hotels open to black patients, and the impact of the Great Depression, which resulted in the closure of the Woodmen of the Union Hospital, the "only available hospital for indigent colored patients in an emergency."[106] Thus, while the ATB believed that it was "performing adequately the service of housing and supporting the transients who are under care at the medical institutions at Hot Springs," its assessment failed to note the ways in which the legalized racism of southern society ensured that comparatively few of these men and women were black.[107]

As diseased men and women descended on Hot Springs, by early 1935 the ATB was providing for four thousand diseased indigents.[108] Unable to cope with a rapidly swelling caseload, Wenger soon found himself having to advise prospective patients *against* a trip to Hot Springs, informing them that the clinic had become so "over-crowded" that it was now necessary to discharge many patients and limit the number of daily admissions.[109] Protesting the ATB's efforts, the inhabitants of Hot Springs resoundingly objected to "the presence of such large numbers of indigent VD cases on the city streets."[110] City officials claimed that many patients were "irresponsible as to their personal conduct"; every day, one local paper reported, twenty-five health seekers faced arrest on charges of drunkenness and disturbing the peace.[111] "If the federal government continues to invite the scum of the earth here," complained a judge to the PHS, "I guess we'll just have to move out and give the town to you."[112]

Hot Springs officials began resisting calls for assistance, even refusing to admit dozens of children whose parents were receiving treatment into the public school system. Despite Wenger's "most vehement protests" and despite repeated assurances that it was "perfectly safe" for these children to mingle with local youth municipal leaders were adamant.[113] They began to push for the removal of the clinic's "undesirable" indigent transients.[114] Acknowledging that "the residents of this city already look with suspicion at persons coming from out of town without resources," federal officials conceded that the PHS clinic was somewhat "justifiably see[n] . . . [as] a menace to their own health, morals, and good reputation."[115]

Conceding that patients "cannot be left to roam at will and get into difficulties on the streets of Hot Springs," federal officials and the ATB considered construction of a camp on the city outskirts to house clinic patients and "give them wholesome occupation and recreation."[116] In addition to responding to local residents' complaints, public officials believed such a facility would lead to significant improvements in standards of care and health outcomes for the city's venereal health seekers. While noting that the policy of purchasing room and board for the clinic's VD patients constituted an improvement over the earlier situation, the executive secretary of the ATB observed that at present, it was "impossible to give proper service with clients scattered over the city."[117] Echoing this, the bureau's director explained that landlords in Hot Springs "do not provide the type of lodging that a sick man should have." "These men are scattered over the city," he continued, "and do not have the supervision needed by venereal people."[118]

Given the fact that since the Depression, many of the city's patients belonged to "a better class of persons," a transient center seemed essential.[119] As the director of the ATB put it: "Many of these people can be reclaimed for society."[120]

Oliver Wenger agreed with this assessment. As he saw it, the practice of housing patients throughout the city was "most unsatisfactory," particularly given the ATB's location "in the negro section of the city." So as to "prevent possible racial friction," Wenger endorsed the government's plan, and in 1934, the ATB began building a camp "for lone men" who were "under care in the United States PHS clinic."[121] From the beginning, this transient center was intended for one group of patients: white men. Wenger's goal was to have the government eventually construct similar camps for African Americans and "single white women," but neither of these plans was ever put into motion.

Camp Garraday opened in 1935. Built on the outskirts of the city in a neighborhood known as the Gorge Addition, the facility's location reinforced contemporary ideas regarding the relationship between VD, poverty, and race. Situated on a thirty-three acre tract of land that was "covered with fine trees," the camp's setting expressed the "natural beauty" of the Ozark mountains.[122] The lone white men housed here encountered a richly financed, state-of-the-art transient center whose amenities included a sixty-bed infirmary, nine barracks, a kitchen, a dining hall, and a recreation building.[123] The surrounding area, which stood in stark contrast with these comparatively luxurious, scenic settings, was occupied primarily by African Americans and "low economic level whites," who lived in "shacks" amid a series of "dilapidated shops" and banks shuttered by the financial crisis that was the Great Depression.[124]

During its first year, the ATB facility quartered five hundred white male transients.[125] While these men—whom Wenger labeled the clinic's "hardest problem"—benefited from the "good food," shelter, immediate medical attention, and recreational opportunities provided directly by the federal government, white women and African Americans of both sexes continued to subsist under the old plan, by which they were "maintained in rooming and boarding houses throughout the city."[126]

Of course, such an arrangement did little to address the most salient obstacles to health for blacks and women. While covering the costs of room and board surely increased their chances of staying within Hot Springs long enough to complete a course of therapy, this program also exposed them to public prejudice and acts of discrimination that a transient camp might have provided shelter from. The fact that both groups on average received fewer shots of Salvarsan than white men *despite not having to pay for hotels or medicines* indicates that matters other than economic ones factored into the differential health outcomes seen at the Hot Springs VD clinic. Though recognizing that these differences could not be explained by way of reference to ignorance or immorality, the PHS was ultimately unwilling to undertake the kinds of environmental reforms (like, for example, hiring black doctors or providing funds to black medical institutions within the city) required to advance the health of women or racial minorities. As a result of this, the PHS's VD control efforts reinforced the racism and sexism the agency sought to combat.

This was the case outside of Hot Springs as well. In 1937, the PHS sponsored an antisyphilis campaign in Georgia that provided testing and treatment services to rural black southerners. Its centerpiece was a mobile clinic unit that traveled roughly five hundred miles every week in search of African American men, women, and children with venereal infections. In addition to running this "Bad Blood Wagon," the campaign issued promotional and educational materials that attempted to draw attention to the structural factors driving the state's exceptionally high rates of syphilis among African Americans. Practically, however, the campaign's approach did not extend beyond doing blood tests and offering shots. Moreover, in his addresses to the public, the white doctor in charge of the clinic issued several remarks about "promiscuity and morality," which, when combined with media images trafficking in "blatant racial stereotypes," significantly hampered the campaign's prospects.[127]

Instead of photographs of sickly patients receiving shots or blood tests, the promotional material released in connection with Camp Garraday consisted largely of depictions of healthy-looking, self-sufficient white men living comfortably within an area made to appear as if it had no association with sickness or clinical services whatsoever. Clean shaven and respectably clad, these individuals appeared in mess halls, kitchens, and outdoor recreation sites without any hint of syphilitic infection. Official reports noted how the camp was located in a "beautiful gorge" and likened the site's "clients" to pleasure seekers, adding that they would derive much benefit from Hot Springs' "desirable surroundings."[128] Striking a sympathetic note, these publications observed that because they were being treated "for serious diseases," the men's ability to contribute to work projects would be "limited."[129]

Camp Garraday embodied the PHS's eugenic understanding of VD. While Wenger labeled white male patients a "problem," they were central to his ideology of "race conservation" and thereby worthy of privileges. Other patients might receive very modest financial aid, but they had to find sources of food and shelter, and they felt the full force of the city's loathing. By contrast, white male

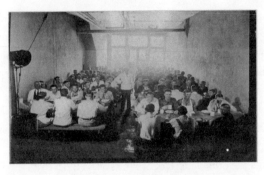

Created for unattached white men, Camp Garraday was situated on the outskirts of Hot Springs. Capable of housing five hundred patients, the camp contained about sixty beds, an infirmary, a recreation center, and—as can be seen in this photograph—a dining facility. Courtesy of the Garland County Historical Society.

patients received care on site, in a domiciliary setting. And Wenger sought to expand the camp's capabilities. In his 1936 budget, he recommended $55,320 for additional forms of support—including a butcher, a recreational supervisor, a housing director, a nursery, and a children's school (with principal and one teacher)—for Camp Garraday's residents.[130]

Wenger's plans never came to fruition. Local white citizens quickly objected, complaining that Camp Garraday, "a Frankenstein monster," restored the "old stigma that Hot Springs is a place only for the treatment of venereal diseases." As the director of the Hot Springs Reservation explained, the PHS's efforts threatened to "ruin the results of the past hundred years of our history, to say nothing of the millions of dollars invested in the resort by private capital." The existence of Camp Garraday functioned to "make the place undesirable for pay patients."[131]

Unable to overcome residents' objections to Wenger's maintenance program and the ATB's camp plan, the federal government terminated the Transient Bureau in 1936 and Camp Garraday ceased to house patients. Venereal health seekers wishing treatment in Hot Springs were required to bring "sufficient funds available to pay their room and board over a period of at least ninety days."[132] For Oliver Wenger, who left Hot Springs in 1937 to take part in Chicago's Syphilis Control Program, it was a bitter ending. It appeared to him that Hot Springs was in no better shape than when he first arrived fifteen years earlier.

The same year Wenger left Hot Springs, Congress passed the National Venereal Disease Control Act. Allotting funds to the states, this legislation enabled a dramatic expansion in the nation's antivenereal infrastructure. Arkansas soon felt the act's effects: prior to 1937 there were no state-run VD clinics here; by 1943, there were eighty-three. These new medical facilities treated fifteen thousand patients per year, far exceeding the numbers treated during the heyday of the Hot Springs VD clinic.[133] In tandem with the mass production of penicillin in the 1940s, these developments led to a precipitous decline in the nationwide incidence of syphilis and gonorrhea. By the early 1950s, the country's VD epidemic had come to an end, and although rates of both syphilis and gonorrhea rose in subsequent decades, the government's model VD clinic played no part in postwar developments.

Conclusion

The history of the Hot Springs VD clinic reveals how eugenics shaped the federal government's response to syphilis and gonorrhea. The facility's day-to-day operations show how the goal of "race conservation" structured patient experiences and outcomes. On account of the high volume of white syphilitics seeking admittance, clinic personnel became increasingly sympathetic to patients' circumstances and needs, and eventually, this sympathy instigated the creation of a medical program that included free treatments as well as stipends for housing and food. While all patients, regardless of race or sex, benefited from these extramedical measures, it is unlikely the PHS would have launched such an approach to VD had not the primary beneficiaries been white males. The Camp Garraday transient center was established to dole out special services to clinic patients who authorities assumed would be white men.

How did eugenics and scientific racism manifest at Hot Springs as compared with Tuskegee? As the failure of its venereological research program suggests, Hot Springs is a story about subjects becoming patients. In Tuskegee, the opposite occurred. What began as a series of mass-treatment campaigns ended up as a horrific forty-year research program revolving around the denial of medical services. Tuskegee's creators tried to explain their complicity by way of reference to the Great Depression, claiming that their actions resulted from agency budget cuts that rendered additional funding for VD treatment impractical. However, the Tuskegee budget cuts appear to be tied to race, because as the Depression deepened, the PHS began pouring money into the Hot Springs clinic, whose patients were provided with drugs as well as with funds for food and shelter. The clientele at Wenger's clinic were primarily white; those enrolled in the Tuskegee study were black.

Race played a determining role in the way the PHS attacked the problem of syphilis and gonorrhea. In broadening the scope of historical study beyond Tuskegee and in particular by looking at the agency's policies toward white patients, we can more clearly see the extent of the government's racialized response to VD. But how did the clinic's existence impact the therapeutic livelihoods of the city's VD specialists? As the next chapter demonstrates, though the PHS's presence in Hot Springs constituted a challenge to resort physicians, it failed to drive them out of the city's venereal marketplace altogether. Instead of abandoning the city to Wenger, local healers maintained a share of the city's shrinking volume in health seekers by overhauling their approach to syphilis.

CHAPTER FIVE

From Hygiene to Hydrotherapy

Private Practitioners in Hot Springs, 1910–1940

On March 10, 1921, a Hot Springs physician named Edward Martin announced that on account of "decreasing patronage," he would be reducing his "office forces" by 30 percent.[1] Over the course of the preceding two decades, Martin had become one of the most successful practitioners in the city, establishing a "large organization" that employed many doctors and nurses.[2] So prosperous did his business become that in 1916, Martin created a "free clinic" within the free bathhouse run by the government, where for several hours each day, he or one of the various members of his staff offered medical services to health seekers unable to afford proper treatment. Unfortunately, these efforts proved unsustainable: in 1920, Martin reported a loss of $5,000 in annual revenue, and the following year brought a further "curtailment of professional business."[3] In response to these setbacks, Martin discontinued his free clinic and fired a number of employees. Despite this, problems persisted. Signaling an inability to practice within Hot Springs any longer, on April 2, 1921, a despairing Martin communicated to city authorities that he would likely soon be "out of it" altogether.[4]

Martin's experience was not unique. Between the 1910s and 1930s, developments both local and global conspired to bring about a "material diminution in the number of bathers" who journeyed to Hot Springs.[5] For one, the appearance of Salvarsan in 1910 threatened to make the treatment of syphilis something that "could be carried out anywhere."[6] Secondly, the creation of the Hot Springs VD clinic in 1921 meant that health seekers who in years past landed in private medical offices such as Martin's clinic were now increasingly availing themselves of the federal government's largesse, receiving free treatment for their venereal ailments.[7] The onset of the Great Depression in 1929 only accelerated these trends, as all across the country, doctors reported increased numbers of syphilitic patients seeking out public medical facilities. For members of the local medical profession, these changed circumstances constituted an existential threat, and they drove many out of business.

Hoping to prevent Hot Springs from becoming a place where people went merely to "spend money and have a good time," resident practitioners rallied around their city's waters.[8] Previously valued for the way they allowed patients to withstand heroic doses of mercury and the iodides of potassium, increasingly, local doctors began to see the springs as a curative substance in their own right, capable of restoring the syphilitic to health even in the absence of these drugs. As standard antivenereal medications fell out of favor, practitioners advocated a straight and simple water cure, arguing that this "Hot Springs effect" was something "no drug or chemical known to science" could replicate.[9] In defense of this position, they advanced two central arguments: that hydrotherapy was a time-tested procedure, one whose value had been certified by eminent medical men of antiquity and whose continuing benefits could be readily seen across the world—especially among the native peoples of the United States, the Philippines, and other Pacific Islands—and that the springs themselves were radioactive, possessing a unique, natural healing agent (radium) that offered an effective, safe cure of syphilis. Taking recourse to medical wisdom both ancient and modern, resort doctors succeeded in holding onto a piece of Hot Springs' shrinking VD marketplace.

The fact that ideas about radioactivity played such a key role in sustaining the resort's popularity during the 1920s and 1930s is telling. In the historical scholarship on medical tourism, the demise of America's turn-of-the-century health resorts is often tied to the appearance of a new class of "magic bullets"—from the chemotherapies of the 1910s through the antibiotic "wonder drugs" of the 1940s and 1950s. According to this narrative, the decline of health seeking was a direct consequence of the laboratory's ever-growing hold over America's therapeutic culture. But the relationship between health seeking and pill popping was more complex than this. As its role in promulgating radium's curative properties shows, instead of being undermined by the advent of modern biomedicine, Hot Springs actually participated in its creation. Neither an antiquated, old-fashioned holdover from premodern times nor a reactionary response to new-fangled therapeutic tools, hydrotherapy was constitutive of modern medical science. Both a product of contemporary developments and a vehicle for the emergence of innovative approaches to illness, the resort's interwar history shows that the tradition of "taking the waters" is neither static nor an oppositional throwback to earlier times.

In large part, what enabled Hot Springs' successful transition from hygiene to hydrotherapy was one of the era's salient medical trends: holism. During the first half of the twentieth century, many Western medical authorities grew dissatisfied with the drift of modern medicine—and in particular with the reductionist styles of thought and practice disciplinary specialization and laboratory science purportedly encouraged. Formalizing a counterhegemonic stance, these doctors labeled themselves "medical holists" and proposed a variety of antireductionist alternatives aimed at broadening medicine's scope.[10] A diverse system of medical thought, holism drew on as many contemporary trends as it rejected; its vision of integrated medical care was at times wholly at odds with modernity and at others quite in line with it. Everywhere it appeared, its development was mediated by regional and local factors.[11]

The healers of Hot Springs participated in this moment of therapeutic reflexivity. In step with their colleagues' growing distrust of mercury and Salvarsan, resort physicians crafted a holistic approach to syphilis, one that demonstrates how widespread the search for "natural" curative methods was in early twentieth-century venereological circles. The popularity of these methods provides an additional context for understanding the Tuskegee study—which Public Health Service (PHS) officials often justified by pointing out how ineffective contemporary medicine's approach to syphilis was. While not at all exonerating the study's founders or minimizing the role that racism played in its creation, this chapter sheds further light on some of the clinical realities that made this experiment thinkable in early twentieth-century America.

The shift from hygiene to hydrotherapy also demonstrates the cultural origins of medical holism in the United States. In their analyses of this movement, historians often contend that American participants in it espoused a narrower version of medical holism than their European counterparts, being concerned primarily with "disciplinary developments" (instead of broader social, political, and cultural phenomena) and embracing "holistic goals through reductionist means" (instead of solutions that went beyond the "technological fix").[12] While the new clinical approach to syphilis that emerged in interwar Hot Springs was in part a response to the threat Salvarsan and the PHS posed to doctors' professional livelihoods, it also played on anxieties of a nonmedical sort—namely, the fear that American men had become "overcivilized." The goal of hydrotherapy as a curative strategy was not only to cure syphilitic bodies but also to preserve white men's patriarchal authority. It promised rejuvenation through connection with the "barbaric virtues" of ancient healers and premodern primitives.[13]

As this suggests, the shift from hygiene to hydrotherapy entailed a realigning of syphilis's moral axes. If late nineteenth-century healers marshaled the "wages of sin" discourse into a therapeutic program designed to protect their white patients from association with (and degeneration into) "amoral" African Americans, their early twentieth-century counterparts turned this project of racial "othering" on its head, using race and morality to create a vision of human sameness linked to long-established tropes of the "noble savage."[14] Throughout this period, local doctors defended Hot Springs' continued relevance by appealing to stereotypes about the virtue and superior wisdom of primitive (often nonwhite) man, whose close proximity to "nature" offered lessons to the "overcivilized" white invalid. Despite the decline of hygienic treatment, ideas about gender, class, and race remained as crucial as ever to local doctors' clinical management of syphilis.

Imperial Origins

If the late nineteenth century witnessed the growth of health resorts within the United States, developments in the early twentieth century played host to the global expansion of American medical tourism. The catalyst for the industry's internationalization was the Spanish-American War of 1898, which resulted in the United States' acquisition of Puerto Rico and the Philippines. Imperialists valued the Philippines for its natural resources and its proximity to the fabled markets of the East and envisioned it as a place that would open the doors to trade with millions of Asian consumers—and thus solve America's overproduction problems.[15] From the beginning of the occupation, however, authorities struggled to attract settlers to this tropical archipelago, as reports of exceptionally high morbidity among US soldiers stationed there threatened to derail plans for economic development on the islands.[16] Some medical authorities believed that white bodies were simply ill equipped for life in the tropics. Others held that the difficulties Americans encountered here were due to environmental rather than racial factors and that therefore adaptation was possible. So as to facilitate the United States' broader economic and geopolitical goals, doctors eagerly sought out means of helping would-be settlers through the process of acclimatization.

Hydrotherapy was critical to this program of climatic adjustment.[17] Early on in the occupation, military observers reported that while malaria and other tropical diseases were endemic to much of the region, the inhabitants of mountainous towns were "better off on account of the natural springs" located therein.[18] Investigations of the Philippine highlands revealed that the islands were home to "numerous hot and mineral springs"—many of which natives believed possessed "remarkable curative properties."[19] After visiting some of these sites and witnessing firsthand the "good results" they yielded in cases of rheumatism, cutaneous ailments, bladder difficulties, and myriad other maladies, military authorities set out to establish a series of health resorts across the islands.[20] Taken together, these curative stations would make long-term residence in the tropics "more comfortable," promoting both "escape" and "recovery" from deadly disease.[21] The hope was that such measures would largely solve "the problem of acclimatization of the white race in the Philippines."[22]

One of the first areas selected for development was Baguio, a highland town located in Benguet province in northern Luzon. Boasting a "pure, cool, invigorating air" and "abundant water," Baguio's climate was likened to that of the Adirondacks, and the colonial government believed that the establishment of sanitariums here would offer relief to those suffering from "diseases prevalent in the lowlands."[23] More to the point, civil authorities contended that Baguio's transformation into a health resort would enable American soldiers stationed in the Philippines to remain in the islands for longer periods of time and thus "reduce the number who go home invalided."[24] The resort was also envisioned as a place that wealthy Filipinos and American settlers might visit; as the area's health infrastructure improved, authorities reasoned, morbidity and mortality rates would plummet, and those considering employment in nearby Manila would no longer feel any apprehension "on account of the climate."[25] As one enthusiastic report put it: "All that is needed to make this place a veritable Mecca during the hot season is railroad transportation."[26] Others hoped that with scientific analysis of these and other springs, the Philippines might become an exporter of "varied and valuable mineral waters."[27]

American dreams of developing Filipino spas and springs appear to have been somewhat unrealistic. While popular travelogues declared that Baguio and other well-known bathing sites possessed "hot springs equal to those in Arkansas," none of the hydrotherapeutic establishments created in the Philippines ever matched the popularity of this famed American health resort.[28] Nevertheless, America's colonization of the Philippines had a lasting impact on medical thought and practice within the United States.

Most notably, imperial conquest generated new interest in the ancient Hippocratic "airs, waters, and places" tradition, which became popular in a variety of Western contexts during the early twentieth century.[29] Despite the emphasis germ theory placed on the bacteriological dimensions of illness, ideas about the connection between environment and health experienced a resurgence during this time, and imperialism was central to the era's incipient neohumoralism. Within colonial locales, theories of acclimatization served as a vehicle for the construction of whiteness and the promulgation of medical policies that discriminated against local populations. Racial matters also factored into the unique brand of environmental determinism that took root within domestic medical

settings, as the movement of Western physicians back and forth between imperial outposts and the metropole facilitated the transfer of ideas, techniques, and
practices from one place to another.[30] The career of a Hot Springs physician
named James C. Minor provides a case in point.

In 1900, shortly after the conclusion of the Spanish-American War, Minor left
his medical practice in Hot Springs and obtained a commission as a surgeon in
the US Army. In his first assignment, he found himself stationed in the Philippines, where he remained until 1903.

Throughout his time here, he toured the islands extensively. On one of his
earliest sightseeing ventures, Minor traveled to the "little valley of Trinidad, province of Benguet," a place that astonished him on account of the boiling hot
streams—"very similar to that of the Arkansas springs"—coursing through its
hillsides.[31] "Naturally interested in the subject of hydrotherapy," Minor was
amazed to learn of these waters' fame, as they were apparently "a favorite with the
natives in the treatment of rheumatic affections and diseases of the digestive organs." The trip impressed on him the value of hydrotherapy.[32]

Encouraged by observations such as these, Minor pioneered a program of hydrotherapeutic research within the US military. His base of operations was the
town of Los Baños, located in the province of Laguna a few hours' ride (by river
steamer) from Manila. "Justly celebrated for its hot springs," Los Baños attracted
a certain amount of attention from civilian tourists, some of whom penned travelogues extolling the "great benefit" they derived from the town's thermal
waters.[33] In the aftermath of the Spanish-American War, Los Baños came to be
valued by the US military primarily on account of its reputation in the treatment
of "scrofulous affections."[34] Shortly after establishing a hospital there, investigators determined that the town's waters were "efficacious for the treatment of syphilis," and with this discovery, the military transformed Los Baños into a site of
venereal therapy.[35] The syphilitic soldiers and sailors treated in Los Baños, authorities claimed, were "easily cured," as the combination of a "moist climate"
and a "high temperature" worked to "eliminate the syphilitic poison from the
system in a manner similar to that exercised by the Hot Springs of Arkansas."[36]
Given this, there could have been no one better positioned to direct the hospital
than James Minor.[37]

Throughout his time as director of the Los Baños Hospital, Minor made "ju-
dicious use of hot baths and vapors," for VD patients as well as those suffering
from other conditions.[38] In one of his first published studies, Minor wrote of an
experiment at Los Baños designed to test hydrotherapy's impact on a group of
soldiers suffering from diseased kidneys. Reporting that "no diuretic [other] than

water was employed," Minor concluded that water alone was sufficient to "bring about the almost normal excretion of urinary solids." On the basis of his findings, presented at a 1902 meeting of the US Army Medical Lyceum in Manila, Minor lambasted the "water abstinence dogma" preached by most military doctors, contending that "much suffering and sickness on the march can be averted by a regulated and uniform use of water externally and internally."[39]

Minor's promotion of hydrotherapeutic cures flowed largely from his overwhelmingly favorable impressions of Filipino health. Everywhere he went, Minor marveled at the general absence of disease and debility among the local population. Speaking of the Igarrotes, for example, he stood in awe of how "few of this hardy race are ever afflicted with disease of any kind."[40] Celebrating the "virtue" of this "primitive" people, Minor linked the relative rarity of tuberculosis, rheumatism, "heart troubles," and other diseases among them to native traditions such as the custom of going about "half naked"—which, among other things, made it easy to obey "calls of nature by simply stepping a pace or two aside" and thus prevented those illnesses consequent on the "prolonged retention of urine." Despite their lack of clothing, Minor observed that syphilis was a "disease unknown" among the Igarrotes, among whom "no case of rape has ever been heard."[41]

Though he praised customary Filipino dress for its positive sanitary effects, Minor glimpsed worrying signs on the horizon. Particularly disturbing were local women who had begun to "imitate the senorita Americana" by donning that "agent of the devil and gynecologists": the corset. "Just how soon the civilizing influence will suggest to the Filipino mother the 'inconvenience' of bearing children," he mused, "remains to be seen."[42] Minor's appraisal of native health often spoke to concerns more germane to the United States than to the Philippines. Raising the specter of "race suicide," his cautioning against the use of corsets reveals a profound ambivalence over the place of the "new woman" within society.

In this, Minor was not alone. Living in an era characterized by the emergence of consumer culture, the closing of the frontier, and women's increased political activism (not to mention that of immigrants and industrial laborers), middle-class white men interpreted developments of the late nineteenth and early twentieth centuries as a challenge to their privileged status as the country's dominant socioeconomic group. As the lower orders aggressively pushed for new rights, and as an older producerist ethos ceded ground to new consumerist values, many came to see themselves as soft—as lacking in virility, as excessively refined urban sophisticates incapable of controlling the "lesser classes" as effectively as their Victorian forebears had.[43] In an attempt to fight off the trend toward overcivilization, leading authorities such as Theodore Roosevelt proposed a variety of revitalizing schemes designed to solve the problem of declining white manhood. Most believed that an injection of "barbarian virtues" was needed, and so arose a cult of primitivism, one that celebrated "authentic" manly values such as physical strength, decisiveness, independence, and courage and that called on effete American brain workers to reacquire these via wilderness excursions, physical activities such as bare-knuckle boxing and football, and the new sport of bodybuilding.[44] Another option, ironically enough, was consumption itself—namely, of the numerous Indian patent medicines marketed by firms such as the Oregon Indian Medicine Company and the Kickapoo Indian Medicine Company.[45] In their own ways, each of these practices promised to restore weakened white men to a place of authority and eminence.

To counter this perceived threat to the country's patriarchal order, Minor prescribed a strong dose of Filipino primitivism. Upon returning to Hot Springs, he became a committed hydropath. In a series of articles bearing titles such as "Water, the Main Factor in the Prevention of Disease" and "Water, the Main Factor in the Treatment of Disease," he spoke of patients who came to Hot Springs because "the latest and most highly approved medication in the treatment of specific diseases" had failed to improve their health.[46] Instead of chemotherapies, Minor championed water as "the first point for the physician and the surgeon to consider in treating any ailment whatsoever."[47] "It is truly marvelous how many disordered conditions of the body can be dissipated by the proper use of water," he exclaimed, drawing particular attention to the role that this simple substance played in enhancing the body's "powers of resistance."[48] For him, "all disease" was a result of "weak resisting power" brought about by the body's failure to flush out continually accumulating toxins. Because ingestion of and immersion in water helped promote "better resisting power," it was the ideal preventive—and therapeutic—agent in any given disease.[49]

Threats

Minor's embrace of water cure brought new levels of attention to hydrotherapy within Hot Springs. Following on his colleague's work, in 1908, a resort physician named Edward Martin published the results of an investigation into the effects of a purely water-based treatment of syphilis on those diseased indigents who made use of the city's free bathhouse. Concluding that the majority of the twenty-five syphilitics he observed were either "improved," "much improved," or "greatly improved" by hydrotherapy, Martin pondered how it was that a venereal disease could be cured "without a dose of medicine."[50]

Others registered similar observations. After examining hundreds of patients who bathed at the free bathhouse, a colleague attempted to explain the benefits water cure offered to the venereally afflicted. Every day, roughly six hundred health seekers took to the springs, most of them "suffering from syphilis of some form and but few receive regular medical attention. The Government bathes these people free, but does not provide medicine or medical service for them. It is gratifying to see the benefits derived from the baths alone in their cases, proving beyond doubt the great beneficial effects of these waters."[51] Inspired by the wondrous performance of the government's "drugless clinic," several doctors began to pursue research into purely hydrotherapeutic approaches to syphilis.

Loyd Thompson was among those impressed with the idea of a "drugless clinic." In a 1917 manual simply titled *Syphilis*, Thompson reiterated decades of accumulated local knowledge about VD therapy. Critical of those who relied "solely upon the specifics" and who totally "disregard[ed] hygienic measures," he argued that the maintenance of "regular" habits, the avoidance of "overwork," and restraint of the "sexual appetite" were essential to the cure of syphilis. In addition to this, Thompson explained how when taken in conjunction with mercury and other antivenereal drugs, the city's waters greatly facilitated recovery from this disease. "The importance of the hygienic treatment of syphilis is hardly to be overestimated," Thompson declared, repeating a refrain that had long been sounded by local medical professionals.[52]

With the passage of time, however, Thompson's hygienic methods gradually transitioned toward something more in line with the therapeutic practices of James Minor and Edward Martin. In an article published in 1931, he relayed the results of an experiment in which he subjected a series of patients to progressively hotter and longer baths. Observing that he was "getting more favorable results than I did before," Thompson concluded that even without mercury or any other drugs, the springs exerted "some favorable action" on syphilis.[53] He attributed this to the "hyperexemia" (or artificial fever) the city's waters induced in his patients.[54] Once committed to hygienic treatment, Thompson now increasingly rooted his curative efforts in hydrotherapy.

By this point, a near consensus had been reached in favor of water cure. After learning of a number of local patients who were "apparently completely cured by the bathing alone," two partners in practice decided to experiment with this method; witnessing hydrotherapy's "striking results," they noted how they "were never able to see such clinical and serological improvements by methods formerly employed, including spinal drainages and the Swift Ellis method."[55] Agreeing with this, a colleague once convinced that the springs merely promoted the "increased elimination" of mercury and other antisyphilitic drugs now shifted course, concluding that the baths themselves were "the most powerful" treatment "in giving good results."[56] Under the new approach, patients were "receiving marked benefit from baths and treatment with less total medication than had been given them before coming for the baths."[57]

The corollary of local doctors' embrace of hydrotherapy was a growing dissatisfaction with contemporary venereology. In 1910, a team of researchers led by the German chemist Paul Ehrlich and the Japanese bacteriologist Sahachiro Hata introduced a new antisyphilitic drug to the world. Dubbed "Salvarsan" and known popularly as "606" (in reference to the fact it was invented only after 605 failed attempts), this arsenical compound quickly acquired the status of a "magic bullet" for syphilis. Indeed, so positive was the American reception of Salvarsan that after severing all commercial ties with Germany during the First World War, the United States government assigned a number of chemical manufacturers the task of devising a home-grown substitute for Ehrlich's drug.[58]

Hot Springs' private practitioners were less sanguine than many of their non-resident colleagues as to Salvarsan's merits. During a 1912 gathering of the Arkansas Medical Society, one local doctor argued that complete reliance on this new drug amounted to "criminal negligence." When a colleague countered this claim, a chorus of Hot Springs physicians interrupted him, voicing their displeasures with "606" and presenting stories of patients disfigured, sickened, and even killed by this new remedy. When one critic opined that "the profession to a large extent are over-enthusiastic about Salvarsan," its lone supporter cheekily retorted that he "[didn't] see anybody around here enthusiastic about it."[59]

The pessimistic reception Salvarsan met with here was largely representative of Hot Springs' more general response to Ehrlich's "magic bullet." While a few lauded "606" as a "wonderful remedy" of "unlimited virtues," most local healers were unfavorably disposed toward the new drug.[60] Their opposition partly owed to Hot Springs' status as the dumping ground of Salvarsan's discontents. Witnessing the travails of syphilitics who came here after having received "one to a dozen shots of '606,'" local healers frequently encountered patients who suffered numerous "complications" resulting from its use.[61] Many came away from these experiences convinced of the drug's dangers and devoted themselves to issuing "little friendly warning[s] as to what may happen in the use of '606.'"[62]

Local practitioners' skepticism toward Salvarsan fed into a more general distrust of this new chemotherapeutic agent—especially in the South. As was the case with resort doctors, some physicians came to distrust Ehrlich's "magic bullet" after witnessing "fatal results" among patients who had been administered this drug within Hot Springs.[63] For others, conversation with local practitioners was enough to generate suspicion.[64] After talking to a "gentleman who practiced medicine in Hot Springs," for example, a doctor in Louisville stopped using the substance and then published an article criticizing colleagues who considered this drug the "last word in syphilis."[65] Praising a resort physician whose practice boasted "the best results from mercury of any man I know," a fellow Kentuckian similarly rejected Salvarsan in favor of older remedies that he believed prevented the disease from reaching its tertiary stage.[66]

In addition to being shaped by their observations of patients "materially injured by the use of arsenic preparations," local doctors' evaluation of Salvarsan was also influenced by professional concerns.[67] Despite their "considerable experience" in treating the "victims" of 606, between the 1910s and 1930s, the popularity of this innovative antisyphilitic medicine steadily eroded the privileged position the city's medical men had long held within America's venereal marketplace.[68] With the arrival of arsphenamine (as Salvarsan was professionally known), outside observers reported that it was now "rare to find a patient who cannot be well taken care of at home."[69] Confirming this, one local practitioner, writing on the eve of America's entry into the First World War, noted how Salvarsan had "so reduced the number of syphilitic patients coming to Hot Springs that . . . the number of baths has fallen off nearly one-third. When one considers," he continued,

> that the syphilitic visitors to Hot Springs were never more numerous than one-half of the total number you can readily see that a loss of one-third of the total number means a reduction of two-thirds of the syphilitic. We see comparatively few cases of secondary syphilis at Hot Springs now, and in fact the largest class of syphilitic patients we have are cerebro-spinal cases who have passed the stage where they are dangerous to the public, but who have also passed the time when a permanent and complete cure can be expected, and who therefore wander from home for treatment.[70]

As Oliver Wenger, the director of the Hot Springs VD clinic, put it: "Since the arsphenamines have justly become popular, the number of syphilitics coming to Hot Springs has been decreased year by year."[71]

With the emergence and spread of Salvarsan, lay and scientific writers began to openly question the resort's therapeutic usefulness. "We have no reason to believe," declared the authors of one medical manual, "that the baths . . . contain appreciable amounts of any medicament that will even indirectly influence the luetic poison."[72] While "a convenient place of retirement for secret treatment" (that is, for patients who wanted to escape friends and family "on account of tell-tale lesions" on exposed parts of the body), the fact remained that "good or better results can be attained elsewhere."[73]

In addition to questioning the effect of the springs on syphilis, an increasing number of physicians adopted a skeptical stance toward the very idea of resort therapy. Some believed that the practice of "taking of waters" was an unproductive pursuit that only encouraged unhygienic modes of life. In a 1913 piece attempting to expose the "humbug of Hot Springs," for example, one medical author lambasted the idea that the water of certain baths and spas contained unique chemical components rendering them more healthful than normal well water. "It is no exaggeration to say," this popular report claimed, "that a gallon of ordinary dish-water with the scum off would have as much curative value as many of our world-famous mineral waters, such for instance as those of Hot Springs of Arkansas."[74] Instead of resting on a scientifically sound foundation, water cure was a product of "religious belief and articles of faith," of mystical notions dating back to mankind's primitive past—when cavemen "worshipped living springs" and visited these sites on account of unwise eating and drinking habits.[75] As such, the practice of "taking the waters" was "ridiculous," "abnormal," and entirely "unwholesome."[76]

All of this contributed to the "local prejudice against Salvarsan" evident within the city.[77] Moreover, as Oliver Wenger himself knew, the PHS's work in Hot Springs constituted a threat to local doctors' professional livelihoods. Cognizant of the fact that the success of his efforts required the cooperation of the local medical profession "more than any other agency," upon his arrival in 1920, Wenger made overtures to members of the Hot Springs Medical Association.[78] The results were not promising. In March 1921, Wenger informed his superiors that he knew of no other VD clinic that was "more liable to criticism from local physicians and others in Hot Springs."[79] Though Wenger was able to acquire the services of a few resident practitioners, the following year, a PHS official observed that "there has been and still exists . . . a feeling among the physicians of the city . . . that the government, in taking patients into the clinic for treatment, is taking fees from them."[80] These sentiments reflected a basic reality of the interwar period, when the PHS's activities in Hot Springs led to a general "curtailment of professional business" for medical doctors. Given this, it is not surprising that they complained of how Wenger had "tak[en] so much work from the regular physician."[81]

Resort doctors found themselves losing business not only because the PHS offered an alternate, free site of treatment for syphilitic men and women but also because the federal government had decided to use the Hot Springs VD clinic as the headquarters for a nationwide educational campaign designed to provide instruction in the treatment of syphilis to medical graduates and established doctors. During the 1920s and 1930s, hundreds of physicians came to Hot Springs as students, enrolling in classes designed to improve their venereological skills. Testifying to the effects of this education, one Mississippi doctor observed how since the clinic's establishment, American physicians now knew "how to handle" venereal diseases better than they "previously did." "We do not need to send them to Hot Springs," this doctor said of his syphilitic patients, adding that as a result of the classes offered at this PHS clinic they were "also able to cure thousands of cases," whereas before they had "many failures."[82] Although clearly beneficial to nonresident healers, local medical men saw this educational endeavor as simply another way in which the federal government was "mak[ing] inroads on their practices."[83]

In addition to these challenges, resort doctors faced the same kinds of obstacles as did doctors all across the country—particularly during the Great Depression. Between 1930 and 1933, the number of individuals who sought out treatment for syphilis or gonorrhea from a privately practicing physician declined by 7 percent. Across the nation, this economic downturn was "in a large measure responsible for the increased number of syphilitics seeking treatment in public clinics."[84] With opportunities for private venereological practice everywhere declining, the future of Hot Springs' status as a sanctuary of the American syphilitic was very much in doubt.

Given this new climate, Hot Springs' resident doctors faced an uphill battle. Recognizing that developments of the early twentieth century threatened to significantly reduce the size of their clienteles, resort doctors faced a professional crossroads: either concede defeat and relinquish their claim to be the country's most skilled VD specialists or find a new way to burnish their venereological credentials. While some chose the former path, many others forged on ahead, and in the effort to maintain Hot Springs as the treatment center par excellence for syphilis, they positioned themselves in opposition to contemporary developments in venereology. In addition to finding fault with Salvarsan, some spoke out against serology, criticizing colleagues who believed that "a positive or negative [Wassermann] quite thoroughly settles the diagnosis and neither history nor previous treatment can weigh in the balance with these magical words."[85] Evincing a clear preference for techniques that appeared "far in advance of laboratory findings," resort physicians marginalized modern medicine's role within the clinic.[86] As one practitioner put it, "We have been too sanguine in our hope that drugs and curative measures" offered the best hope for syphilitic patients.[87]

Holism and Hydrotherapy

In critiquing doctors who placed too much faith in "drugs and curative measures," the healers of Hot Springs aligned themselves with one of the interwar
period's leading medical developments: holism. In the aftermath of the Great
War, a number of leading Western intellectuals developed a profound skepticism
toward science and medicine. Concerned that the costs of technological progress
outweighed their benefits, a growing chorus of medical and scientific professionals argued that the war's unfathomable death tolls were directly related to science's increasingly reductionist outlook, contending that the invention of poison
gas, machine guns, and other forms of industrial weaponry were a direct result
of the trend toward laboratory research. At the same time, the unthinkable mortality rates of the 1918–19 influenza pandemic prompted mass criticism of doctors and health care professionals, and indeed, many medical workers saw their
inability to prevent the spread of this deadly virus as evidence of the laboratory's
inefficacy.[88] These pessimistic currents prompted a great deal of soul searching
within medicine, the end result of which was a newfound level of appreciation
for earlier traditions, which—in contradistinction to contemporary trends—were
believed to stress individual physiological uniqueness, the social, material, and
environmental dimensions of health and illness, and the body's natural healing
powers.[89]

While these tendencies had been present within Western medicine for centuries, World War I lent them institutional and professional support, as now, self-
styled "holists" consciously positioned them in opposition to mainstream medicine. In medical books and journals, research institutes, university courses, and
a variety of professional fora, holists developed a scathing critique of contemporary
biomedicine, proposing new, antireductionist ways of understanding the body
and securing its health.

For holists, the watchword of the day was integration. Believing that modern
medicine had erred in splitting up the body into its component parts, holists
strove to treat their patients as individuals—as people whose illnesses resided not
in diseased organs or tissues, but in the body and mind more generally. Such an
approach necessitated the unifying of medicine's increasingly fragmented sub-
fields, which were synthesized under new, generalizing rubrics such as "biopsy-
chosocial" and "constitutional" medicine.[90] And instead of prioritizing the laboratory and its scientific methods of diagnosis, holists stressed the importance of
bedside observation, presenting medicine as an art that required intuition more
than technical expertise. Along with their penchant for individualized interpre-

tations of illness, holists argued that the best forms of therapy were "natural"—
that is, those that aided the body's own efforts to recover health.[91]

In order to legitimize their critique of orthodox medicine, holists turned to
Hippocrates, whose image they transformed into a symbol of antimodernism.
Embracing the therapeutic wisdom of ancient Greece, holists presented themselves as "plain men" who valued tradition. They implored their colleagues to
work with nature instead of against it and to seek the solutions to contemporary
medical problems in the distant past.[92] Yet despite their appeals to ancient authority, those who participated in the interwar period's "Neo-Hippocratic" movement accepted as much of modernity as they rejected. When invoking the Hippocratic text *Airs, Waters, and Places*, for example, they did so in defense of both
humoral and mechanistic thinking.[93] Moreover, many holists reserved a place for
the laboratory within their visions of integrated care, making use of analytical,
reductionist methodologies even as they criticized others who did so. Instead of
being an internally consistent system of alternative medical thought, holism was
diverse, mediated by local factors everywhere it appeared.[94]

Particularly pronounced were the differences between the American and European branches of this interwar medical movement. In comparing these, historians have generally found the former to be "meliorist" in orientation, lacking
the strident antimodernism and broader social and political aspects of European
responses to the era's crisis in medicine. Within the United States, medical authorities such as George Robinson (dean of Vanderbilt University's School of
Medicine and author of the 1939 book *The Patient as a Person*), Walter Cannon
(chair of Harvard Medical School's Physiology Department and author of the 1932
text *The Wisdom of the Body*), and Alan Gregg (medical services director of the
Rockefeller Foundation) sought to counter the trend toward disciplinary specialization, to encourage greater study of the nonphysical factors influencing individual health, and to deemphasize the use of drugs in medical therapy. Yet despite their calls for a holistic approach to medicine, for each of these men,
antireductionism was generally a clinical and professional matter. Instead of
extending their critique to broader social, economic, or political phenomena,
American holists placed the burden of adjustment to modern life squarely on patients' shoulders.[95] Only European holists, most historians agree, sought something more radical than a mere accommodation to modernity.

While this interpretation captures the views of holism's leaders, historians
have yet to paint a broader picture of the movement's development in specific local contexts, and among nonelite healers. During the 1920s and 1930s, the era's
holistic currents spread through the community of medical practitioners active

in Hot Springs, which already had an uncomfortable relationship with modern medicine. Speaking to this, in 1893, one local practitioner delivered an address to the American Medical Association that set out to correct the "monstrous dictum . . . that the medical practice of our fathers did more harm than good." While respecting the "genius of Pasteur" and the era's other "wonderful advances," this doctor contended that there was much of value to be found in the "medical literature of the past." In studying practices that dated back to "remotest antiquity," he argued, the profession might better "navigate with increased safety amid the rocks and reefs and along the siren shores of our modern age of constant revolution and change."[96]

Developments of the early twentieth century reinforced these sentiments. Tossed about by the invention of Salvarsan and the creation of the Hot Springs VD clinic, the city's medical men navigated their way through "our modern age" by fully embracing holistic teachings. Like their counterparts elsewhere, local healers did this in part by invoking the medical traditions of Greco-Roman antiquity. As one resident physician declared, far from being a "hit or miss shotgun treatment," hydrotherapy was ancient, something whose use "dates back to the time of Hippocrates and has been employed by some of the most eminent physicians of every period."[97]

Physicians in early twentieth-century Hot Springs leaned heavily on the medical wisdom of the ancients. Drawing on biblical accounts of lepers and syphilitics bathing in the "various pools and rivers" of the ancient Middle East and on Latin texts recounting the "magnificent" hydrotherapeutic structures of the Roman Empire, they presented Hot Springs as a contemporary analogue of long-lost baths and spas, replete with all their "marked healing power."[98] Of particular importance was the Hippocratic treatise *Airs, Waters, and Places*, which one local healer termed "the best account we have of the use of water in various forms in the treatment of disease in the early history of medicine." Observing that "since the days of Hippocrates and Galen, water had been used as a curative agent for all diseases," resort doctors relied on this volume to establish "the present day value of thermal baths in the treatment of syphilis."[99]

Statements such as these played directly into the controversy over the origins of syphilis. Although most paleopathologists today agree that this disease was confined to the New World until Columbus's voyages across the Atlantic during the 1490s, in the early twentieth century pre-Columbian theories were in ascendance.[100] Countering the claim that the Americas were "the cradle of syphilis," local practitioners argued that this venereal malady had its origins "in the dim recesses of antiquity." Their embrace of the "airs, waters, and places" tradition was accompanied by a belief that syphilis existed in the Old World "[well] before the sailing of Columbus."[101] Citing various "historic records" demonstrating how ancient Hebrew and Graeco-Roman peoples "made use of water" in the treatment of "leprosy, syphilis, and the more common skin disorders," local physicians saw themselves continuing a form of venereal therapeutics that had been practiced "since the dawn of our present civilization."[102] "Syphilis is one of the ancient diseases," one of the city's medical men proclaimed and as such was "susceptible" (or receptive) to all of the "environmental factors" discussed in the works of "older writers."[103]

Members of the local medical profession also turned to the ancient past when arguing for the positive effect hydrotherapy had on patients' mental states. Recognizing that the pain brought on by syphilis had "a very destructive effect on the brain and its mental processes," resort doctors believed that the successful treatment of disease required an attention to what one termed "mental prophylaxis."[104] On account of their "very decided psychological effect," the city's waters met this requirement.[105] In defense of this claim, local healers pointed to the past. "The Roman visitor in search of health," two local physicians reminded their colleagues, "read these lines as he approached the baths of Caracassa": "Light of heart approach the shrine of health, / So shalt thou leave with body freed from pain. / For here's no cure for him who is full of care."[106] A robotic and "machine-like" discipline, modern medicine overlooked the "mental attitude" of the patient, fixating solely on "powders and potents." Distancing themselves from this, resort physicians sought to prevent "the loss of that 'art' of psychotherapy" and used the city's waters to help health seekers "regain a new hold on life."[107]

Like holists more generally, Hot Springs doctors expressed a desire to recover the lost knowledge of the "olden days," when men and women knew "the value of the fever process."[108] Agreeing that previous generations of venereal health seekers had "received benefits beyond that obtained during the last twenty or thirty years," local healers concluded that it was "necessary to have [the baths] given quite differently from what had been the custom for many years."[109] Whereas previously, doctors aimed to avoid any "undue discomforts or consequences," the hydrotherapeutic approach to syphilis followed a different directive: "Give as much rise of temperature as the patient would tolerate."[110]

Eschewing convenience, hydrotherapy was a deliberately discomforting curative method. Loyd Thompson, for example, noted that the first patients he administered the water cure to were "mighty sick . . . for a while."[111] Commenting on the effects of hydrotherapy, a colleague remarked that this effectively transformed chronic conditions into acute ones—which typically ended either in "rapid recovery or death."[112] While perhaps an exaggeration, it bears noting that water-induced fatalities were not entirely unknown to Hot Springs. One case involved a local physician with chronic interstitial nephritis. Taking to the waters following a banquet at which he ate and drank "freely," this individual's temperature eventually reached 107 degrees Fahrenheit. "Capillary hemorrhages occurred all over the body," a medical report stated. "He passed away in violent convulsions, the body a blackened mass. The temperature after death was 112 degrees."[113]

As a curative method, hydrotherapy was valued for its ability to "shock" the patient's body into action, and the effect of this was often quite violent. Indeed, according to local practitioners, it was relatively common for patients in other places to "discontinue treatment" on account of the "intensity" of the reaction.[114] In its own studies, the PHS determined that a bath temperature of over 105 degrees Fahrenheit frequently yielded "certain ill effects"—namely, heat exhaustion.[115] Of particular concern were female patients, some of whom reportedly "faint[ed]" or came away with "very severe headaches."[116]

Despite these dangers, resort physicians believed the hydrotherapeutic cure of syphilis superior to other, drug-based measures. In defending the value of the city's waters, they often pointed to an earlier era in the city's history. "Remarkable results were obtained back in the old days," one physician explained, "before bath houses were built, by patients remaining in the hot water until a marked reaction was produced rather than by taking a more comfortable bath, as has been principally used during the past twenty-five years. The change from the old manner of taking the baths to that of the present date was probably brought about largely by the public demanding that they be treated without being made so uncomfortable as in the development of a high fever which takes place when one is immersed in our hot water for any considerable time."

Though uncomfortable, this "old manner of taking the baths" constituted "the greatest aid we have to offer in the treatment of syphilis."[117] Concurring with this, a colleague recalled how "years ago we had what was vulgarly known as the 'Old Raal Hole,'"—a pool of water frequented by paupers of all types. Initially wading into cooler parts of the pool, patients gradually made their way toward "hotter and hotter" water. "In many instances," this physician recalled, individuals suffering from "syphilitic skin lesion[s]" were healed "as if by magic without any medication whatsoever."[118]

As its potentially unwelcome consequences indicate, the hydrotherapeutic treatment of syphilis was part of the era's craze for "barbarian" medical therapies. The scholarship on American holism contends that this was a purely professional movement lacking any broader cultural foundation, but the evidence from Hot Springs indicates that fears of overcivilization lurked not too far beneath the surface of holistic medical practice. Indeed, it is for this reason that doctors' primitivist prescriptions were defended by way of reference to the medical traditions of numerous "savage" peoples. As one doctor put it, "Hydrology in its various phases has been practiced by the primitive tribes and races of the world practically from the beginning of time."[119]

Among these tribes were Native Americans. According to local healers, hydrotherapy was a central part of the continent's indigenous medical traditions. Testifying to this, one resort doctor wrote of his experience "among the Indians of the western frontier," where

> I found their principal medicinal agent to consist of the "Sweating Tepee," which was regarded as a sovereign remedy among the various tribes occupying the northern border. . . . The patient entered the teepee through a small opening near the ground, covered with a flap, armed with a jar of water, which was thrown upon the rocks, and remained for twenty or thirty minutes, or until a full stage of perspiration had been reached. And now, thoroughly relaxed, the patient plunged into a nearby stream in order to secure the cold shock. This method of cure was common among the Sioux and other northern tribes and was carried on . . . with most excellent results.[120]

According to this author, Indian forms of hydrotherapy were particularly effective in cases of rheumatism, neuritis, and the common cold.

By the late nineteenth century, the folklore surrounding Hot Springs' early history was chock full of stories about Indians—whom most credited with the region's discovery.[121] As local authorities had it, long before Europeans arrived on the continent, tribes native to the area had discovered the springs' healing powers. According to most of these mythic tales, Native Americans had an "unlimited faith" in these waters and believed that their "Great Spirit" resided in them.[122] During the early twentieth century, commentators began to attribute the springs' alleged popularity among Native Americans to syphilis. As one local doctor had it, "Knowing the high percentage of syphilis existing in the Indians of North America," it was "not difficult to imagine that they not only needed the baths of Hot Springs, but received much benefit from them."[123]

Local healers also drew parallels between their practices and those of Pacific Islanders. Speaking to the value of "heat therapy," two resort doctors observed how on the island of Java, "the natives undertake to cure syphilis by bathing in the waters of the hot springs." Crouching or reclining near the springs, patients used the shell of a coconut or a "hollow bit of bamboo" to pour hot water "regularly and continually" upon their sores—usually for many hours at a time. After a few weeks of this treatment, syphilitic Javanese men and women were capable of bringing about "complete cures of external lesions."[124]

As these remarks indicate, occupational obstacles like those faced by Hot Springs' private practitioners contributed to the general sense of decline that set in among many white middle-class professional men during the early twentieth century. Facing problems that were at once professional and sociocultural, Minor and his colleagues responded by crafting a form of venereal therapeutics that addressed both the threat to their livelihoods and the perceived threat to their status. Tying together the early twentieth century's "crisis in medicine" and its "masculinity crisis," the hydrotherapeutic response to syphilis aimed to restore the venereally afflicted not only to health but also to a sense of lost manhood—both for doctor and patient. It is perhaps for this reason that local doctors cautioned against water's use in the treatment of female health seekers, who were apparently unable to withstand the effects of the fever process. Through partaking in a therapeutic procedure linked to strong, active, powerful "savages," syphilitic white men of the early twentieth century could regain their place as the nation's dominant socioeconomic force.

Radium, Heat Therapy, and the Search for "Natural" Cures

Articulating their resort's relevance by way of reference to ancient hydrotherapeutic sources offered definite benefits to local healers. But Neo-Hippocratic thought only supported the concept of hydrotherapy in a general sense. So as to attract patients to Hot Springs specifically, resort therapists needed to counter the claim that "all waters will act the same way if administered alike."[125] Of particular importance in this context were studies documenting the presence of radioactive materials in the city's waters, to which local doctors quickly attached a holistic meaning.

Among members of the American scientific community, the question of the springs' specific chemical contents had long been a subject of debate. Responding to calls that it undertake a scientific examination of the city's waters, in 1905 the federal government sent two chemists to the region, and their investigations revealed that the springs possessed decidedly radioactive properties.[126] Following up on this, a 1916 study conducted by a University of Missouri chemist revealed that the average quantity of radium in the waters of Hot Springs was .45 millimicrocuries (or 1.24 mache units)—a level of radioactivity that "correspond[ed] favorably with certain well known European springs."[127]

In the wake of these findings, local healers began conducting their own analyses, all of which attributed the "remarkable and peculiar effects" seen among the city's ailing bathers to radioactivity. The implications were obvious; as one resident physician pronounced, those doctors who advised their patients to "take hot baths at home instead of going to Hot Springs" misunderstood the "true physiological effect of these waters," as their uniquely radioactive nature meant that there was something "peculiar to [this] place."[128] "In the absence of any other reason," a colleague concurred, "we are compelled to give to radioactivity the cures which the people do not get from ordinary water."[129]

Thus was the mystery of the "Hot Springs effect" solved: instead of benefiting from "rest" or "change of scene," it was radium that explained these waters' magical healing properties. As one study concluded, a bath in the city's waters raised an individual's body temperature "very promptly in a few minutes to 101, 102, 103, and even to 105 degrees Fahrenheit"—an effect that "ordinary water, no matter how hot," could not reproduce.[130] Accompanying this rise in body temperature were a host of other physiological changes associated with amplified cellular activity, from increased heart rate to decreased blood pressure—along with profuse perspiration and urination.

Throughout the 1920s and 1930s resident practitioners persistently highlighted the antisyphilitic powers of the city's radioactive waters. Responding to those who believed its waters "not unique in activity," doctors pointed to the thousands of "invalided people" who annually sojourned in Hot Springs just to experience their "peculiar therapeutic value." "The remarkable values in the hot water of this reservation," one physician explained, "lie chiefly in the potency of the water's radio-emanation."[131] For the diseased, Hot Springs' radioactive waters promised "renewed vitality," and the "increased metabolic rate or cell change" the waters promoted quickly became a selling point for local practitioners—even those who used them in conjunction with mercury and Salvarsan.[132]

Local healers' attempt to position radioactivity as the key to the springs' antisyphilitic prowess was much more than a therapeutic shot in the dark. Over the course of the early twentieth century, the discoveries and inventions of Marie Curie and Ernst Rutherford encouraged doctors to explore the medical effects of radium, and as a result, the use of this radioactive element in the treatment of cancer, syphilis, and a variety of other conditions gained widespread acceptance.[133] So too did the idea that Hot Springs exuded a radioactive essence, as many leading scientific voices attributed these waters' "apparent therapeutic virtues" to their "radium-impregnated" nature.[134] The discovery of this "wonderful natural healing agent" therefore provided local physicians a new selling point, something they could use to lure prospective venereal health seekers to this central Arkansas resort.[135]

Bolstered by these new discoveries, local healers devised a new, multipronged curative routine, one that yoked the springs' radioactive properties to a full complement of existing hydrotherapeutic delivery systems. The process began in the bathhouse, where for between five and twenty minutes each day, patients soaked in a tub of water heated to a temperature of 96 to 100 degrees Fahrenheit. Direct contact with the "fresh radio-active spring water" allowed the skin to be "penetrated by the various rays" of radium, which stimulated body cells and facilitated the elimination of waste products and toxins.[136] From here, bathers moved into a vapor cabinet, where they inhaled emanations of radium that promoted the retention of radioactive material within the lipoid tissues of the lungs. Their vital organs thoroughly excited, patients then had towels saturated with hot water applied to their backs, which caused the molecules of radium to begin to break down and disintegrate within their bodies. In the final step, patients imbibed large quantities of hot water, which permitted "the administration of larger amounts of radium emanation, and add[ed] to the effects of that absorbed during the other procedures of the bath."[137]

The end result of this hydrotherapeutic regimen was something local doctors termed the "cure reaction."[138] The value of radium therapy lay in its ability to restore the "vital energy of growth and repair" naturally lost by body cells and tissues through aging. Leading to an "increased feeling of strength and rejuvenation," it literally shocked these into action, "making them perform their proper function."[139] If such a procedure was not guided, a "violent reaction" might ensue.[140] This is why travel to Hot Springs yielded superior results in comparison with treatment with water "artificially made radio-active."[141] As one resort physician noted: "The effects derived from the Hot Springs thermal waters are not wholly due to its radioactive properties, but are due as well to the careful and regulated application of these thermal waters to the body."[142]

The city's doctors incorporated radium into a holistic defense of the virtues of the waters of Hot Springs. As did holists elsewhere, local medical men subscribed to a belief in the body's innate disease-fighting capacities, contending that "the individual is well equipped with a natural pharmacopeia perfectly capable of coping with and overcoming the majority of diseases."[143] Because on this view sickness was the result of "weak resisting power," the healers of Hot Springs concentrated their efforts not on the "annihilation of organisms sometimes acting as bearers of disease" but instead on helping their patients maintain a "normal power of resistance."[144] In this holistic endeavor, the "mysterious forces of nature" known as X-rays were of inestimable value.[145]

The discovery of Hot Springs' radioactive properties was not the only medico-scientific development of the early twentieth-century that factored into local healers' promotion of water cure. While the popularity of radium therapy offered them a means of countering the threats posed by Salvarsan and the PHS, so too did "heat therapy"—a curative procedure whose origins date back to the experiments of a German doctor named Julius Wagner-Jauregg. In 1927, Wagner-Jauregg announced a new means of combating syphilis: malaria.[146] Based on the idea that the parasites responsible for this disease possessed antivenereal properties, malaria therapy fired the imaginations of researchers during the 1920s and 1930s, and their experiments with this stimulated dozens of new approaches to syphilis. Most aimed to avoid the high mortality rates associated with Wagner-Jaurreg's technique—that is, to devise an alternative to this that "would have the same therapeutic effect as malaria but with less attendant danger."[147] Eventually, it became clear that the success of the Wagner-Jauregg method had less to do with malaria than with this disease's symptoms—namely, fever. Thus was born the idea of "artificial fever therapy," also known as "heat therapy."[148]

Like other physicians, Hot Springs' medical practitioners eagerly experimented with malaria therapy. In 1930, Loyd Thompson published the results of his own experience with this innovative procedure, concluding that he was "sold on the subject of malarial inoculation."[149] Most believed that while "satisfactory in many cases," the mortality rate associated with the Wagner-Jauregg method was "too high" for use among any but the most skilled practitioners.[150] Quite naturally, local doctors offered the springs as a substitute for malaria therapy, contending that the radioactivity of the city's waters lent them a fever-producing power far superior to that seen elsewhere. Boasting a "relatively safe" and "more economic" form of fever therapy, local doctors argued that Hot Springs was clearly the nation's "greatest available asset" in the treatment of syphilis.[151]

For resident physicians, the appeal to modern, cutting-edge laboratory science constituted one means of currying the favor and patronage of prospective venereal health seekers. That such methods produced the desired results can be seen in the reports of southern health departments, which regularly noted instances of syphilitic patients being "sent to Hot Springs, Arkansas for fever therapy."[152] Those referred here received daily baths for four to six weeks, during which their average body temperatures reached around 103 degrees Fahrenheit.[153] Whether or not these were combined with regular injections of Salvarsan, mercury, and bismuth, doctors found that the new hydrotherapeutic technique led to greatly improved outcomes. "We have obtained better results since we have been using fever baths," one team of doctors observed, adding that these patients "have been symptom free and serologically negative after two years on this line of treatment."[154]

In elevating "natural" therapies over chemical ones, resort doctors were not alone. Nor were they the only healers to offer a holistic critique of modern venereology or to opine that syphilis was a "self-limited disease."[155] During the interwar period, medical researchers at various universities began to analyze clinical data from VD patients treated at hospitals and clinics all across the country, and their findings often called into question both the safety and efficacy of mercury, arsphenamine, and other standard antisyphilitic medications. Pointing to evidence suggesting it might be capable of "spontaneous" cure, specialists published articles such as "Recovery from Severe Syphilis without Medicine" and recounted stories of patients who forsook "ordinary treatment" and instead took up courses of "diet and baths."[156] Looking not only at germs but also at the "soil" in which germs developed, medical authorities increasingly directed their efforts toward improving the condition of "the host."[157] As one practitioner put it: "The healing power of nature is often sufficient to combat the double task of overcoming the disease as well as its orthodox treatment."[158]

The first step in assisting nature's "healing power" was to refuse to administer "poison[s]" such as Salvarsan to syphilitic patients.[159] Opinions varied as to the next step. Some doctors turned to electricity and various "combination drugless treatments."[160] For others, the solution was hydrotherapy. Indeed, far from being limited to Hot Springs, this alternative approach to venereal therapeutics found favor among a number of nonresident physicians. Defending his decision to employ "measures other than the usual medicinal remedies," one physician in Wabash, Indiana, administered a course of "twenty-one sweat baths in a hot-air oven" to all his syphilitic patients. "I have yet to find a case of syphilis," he reported, "who has had a recurrence of the disease in any form whatever. I have never found it necessary to resort to medication of any kind, irrespective of the condition of the patient. They have come to the office with pustular eruptions, chancres and the other usual syphilitic eruptions and in from two to four weeks all traces have disappeared."[161] The length of time required to produce a hydrotherapeutic cure of syphilis, this doctor reported, was "shorter than with the routine mercury-potassium-iodide method in general use today."

Endorsements of venereological holism such as these often bore the mark of Hot Springs' influence. In a 1927 debate sponsored by the *Kentucky Medical Jour-*

nal, one local doctor seized the floor and asked his colleagues, "What cures syphilis?" Responding to his own query, he then went on to declare that while mercury and Salvarsan might prove useful adjutants to the disease's cure, by themselves, "none of these drugs will cure syphilis."[162] In the end, only the "body itself" could affect this.[163] Concurring with this, a colleague then reiterated that "we do not cure syphilis with any of the so-called antisyphilitic drugs."[164] Rather, "the body cures itself"; medications act only to stimulate the body's natural healing processes.[165] Worried that his audience had perhaps not heard these words clearly enough, this physician then declared: "Syphilis should never be treated[,] . . . but the patient should be handled." And when it came to how to best handle the patient, the best place to start was "in diet, in exercise, in fresh air, and in that most powerful antisyphilitic remedy: hydrotherapy."[166]

Interestingly, even those who reserved a place for Salvarsan and mercury noted how "more and more, to the great advantage of patients, physicians are beginning to employ thermal cures in the treatment of syphilis."[167] After reading a paper by two Hot Springs doctors, a pair of physicians at the Kansas City General Hospital conducted an experiment in which syphilitic patients were treated "by means of hot baths in an ordinary bath tub."[168] Even though their city's waters were entirely lacking in radioactivity or "other mysterious elements," the results of this study were promising and led the pair to conclude that "all individuals, no matter what their type of syphilis . . . would benefit by a course of these baths."[169] Experiments such as these stimulated an awareness among doctors all across the country that antisyphilitic pyrexia could be induced "by prolonged hot baths either in the house, hospital, or at hot springs."[170] Admitting that "for many years better results were secured at Hot Springs than any other place," a venereologist in Nebraska advised his readers to replicate the city's hydrotherapeutic methods, as heat worked to raise the syphilitic patient's immunity and thus made chemical remedies "twice as effective."[171]

Even the PHS expressed an interest in hydrotherapy. In the late 1920s, Oliver Wenger began a series of experiments at the Hot Springs VD clinic designed to test water cure's efficacy "as an adjunct to the treatment of syphilis."[172] Over the course of six weeks, thirty of the study's subjects received regular injections of Salvarsan and mercury in conjunction with a daily hydrotherapeutic regimen consisting of a fifteen-minute bath. A second, smaller group of nine subjects entered the bathhouse everyday but received "no medication of any kind."[173] Gradually, the temperature of the water administered in these baths was increased, beginning at 100 degrees Fahrenheit and raised to 105 degrees Fahrenheit during the final week of the study. The results showed that while recipients of the "combined therapy" demonstrated a "rapid reversal of the Wassermann reaction," such was not the case for those not given any antisyphilitic drugs. As Wenger put it: "Hydrotherapy alone has no marked influence on the course of the disease, since the Wassermann findings remained unchanged and secondary manifestations persisted longer than in the first group."[174]

The fact that the federal government conducted research on the efficacy of drugless antisyphilitic protocols is incredibly significant, especially in light of the Tuskegee study. Wenger's hydrotherapeutic experiments suggest that like academic venereologists, the PHS's VD Division did not know what the optimal treatment for syphilis was and was willing to entertain theories that it was self-limited. Indeed, even though the results of this research indicated that water cure was comparatively ineffective, the very undertaking of such an investigation reveals an openness to "natural" approaches to syphilis on the government's part. A similar curiosity likely factored into the design of the Tuskegee study, even if this reveals little about the racist attitudes that shaped its origin and execution. Like doctors all across the country, PHS officials conceived this experiment at a time in which the belief that syphilis was "curable . . . without drugs, serums, or salves" represented a growing consensus within interwar American medicine.[175]

Conclusion

Early twentieth-century doctors promoted travel to central Arkansas for many of the same reasons as their nineteenth-century counterparts. As in days past, they pointed to the "greater advantage" of resort-based therapy, arguing that in Hot Springs "the entire time could be given over to the treatment, sans business, friends, etc., plus elimination, before, during, and after."[176] At times channeling a neurasthenic discourse, they reiterated earlier ideas about the "renewed vitality" that accompanied travel to the region, as those with "brains be-fogged," muscles dammed with the "unexpected products of wines and trimmings," and nervous systems "burned in the mid-day fury of a Wall Street" could all be "cleared and made good as new by the waters of Hot Springs."[177]

With the passage of time, however, hygienic treatment fell out of favor. Speaking to this, in an address delivered to the Mississippi Valley Medical Association in 1911, James C. Minor proclaimed that "two subjects" dominated the outside world's conception of Hot Springs: "water and morality." "Being a student of the physical," he continued, "I prefer to talk of water." According to Minor, it was with "the physical, not the moral[,] side of life" that doctors had to concern themselves, as the aim of medicine was "physical perfection."[178]

Minor's remarks effectively illustrate one part of Hot Springs' therapeutic evolution from the late nineteenth to the early twentieth century. With the advent of hydrotherapy, the "moral therapy" of an earlier era was displaced, and attempts to cure syphilis fixated solely on the physical body. Once taught that their illnesses were the result of sinful lifestyles desperately in need of correction, patients now were treated by doctors concerned primarily with the action of radium molecules and the monitoring of bodily temperatures. Instead of anchoring their efforts in behavioral modification, resort physicians now sought to modify the interior environment of the syphilitic body.

Yet while hydrotherapy may have neglected the moral side of life, it involved much more than the physical cure of syphilis. Nurtured by fears of overcivilization, water cure spoke to status-conscious white, middle-class American men troubled by the challenges women, blacks, immigrants, and industrial laborers posed to the traditional social order. Linked to the health customs of hardy, aggressive, strong-willed "primitives," it offered beleaguered patriarchs hope for the restoration of older systems of racial and sexual domination. Likening the baths to an injection of "barbarian virtues," resort physicians marshaled hydrotherapy into the service of social, political, and cultural hegemony. In doing so, they crafted a version of medical holism that was very different from the narrow-minded, clinically oriented, "reductionist" version of this movement in other parts of the United States. Built on contemporary cultural attitudes every bit as much as "moral therapy" was during the nineteenth century, hydrotherapy enabled resort doctors to hold onto a portion of the city's dwindling market in venereal health seekers—thus ensuring that Hot Springs' status as a syphilitic asylum would survive well into the twentieth century.

Epilogue

On July 15, 1949, Mrs. J. C. Reynolds of Port Neches, Texas, sent a letter to the director of her state's health department. Addressing recent developments in public health, Reynolds explained that while traveling through the neighboring state of Arkansas on a recent vacation with her husband, she had "noticed several billboards along the highway calling attention to the syphilis menace" as well as numerous "mobile units"—traveling clinics that moved from town to town offering the state's residents "free blood tests" for syphilis. Remarking on "the good which could be accomplished through such actions as these," Reynolds pondered why it was that other states had "not become more concerned over this menace to society," noting that on returning home she was reassured that "Texas is not going to lag behind in this important matter."[1]

Reynolds's observations highlight some of the ways the United States' response to syphilis changed over the course of the 1930s and 1940s. Aiming to combat the "hush-hush attitude toward the subject of venereal disease," throughout these decades the country's medical and political leaders intensified their efforts to control the spread of syphilis and gonorrhea, maladies said to have attained "epidemic" proportions in the wake of the Great Depression and the Second World War.[2] The origins of this ramped-up disease-control campaign date to President Franklin D. Roosevelt's second term, a period in which Congress passed both the Social Security Act (1936) and the National Venereal Disease Control Act (1937). While the former made funds available for grants-in-aid to states for "all phases of public health work," the latter allotted funds specifically for the control of syphilis and gonorrhea.[3] As a result of these federal expenditures, by the time Mrs. Reynolds wrote her letter commending Arkansas's "Have You Got Syphilis?" billboards, the American incidence of venereal disease had begun a precipitous decline—one that continued throughout the early 1950s.

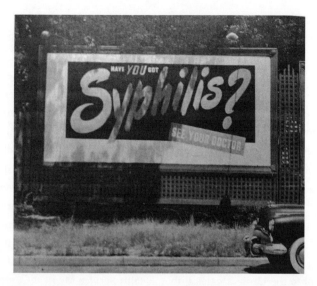

Published in the *Arkansas Health Bulletin* (6:8 [1949]: 3), the caption to this photograph of Arkansas's "Have You Got Syphilis?" billboard explains that "the special education project of the VD Division using billboards and car cards to get people to seek blood tests is attracting considerable attention. The large letters on the black background are a startling shade of red, which some Health Department employees have called *syphilis pink.*"

Arkansas's experience was representative of how states responded to the federal government's renewed antivenereal efforts. Prior to 1937, the only governmentally sponsored medical facility dedicated to the diagnosis and treatment of syphilis and gonorrhea within this southern state was the Hot Springs VD clinic, operated by the Public Health Service (PHS). Yet after the passage of the aforementioned pieces of legislation, Arkansas's antivenereal infrastructure rapidly expanded; by 1943, the state was home to eighty-three VD clinics, which together treated roughly fifteen thousand venereal cases per year.[4] In addition to dramatically increasing its clinical capabilities, the state's health department also created a VD control registry and embarked on an ambitious public relations campaign designed to spark awareness of syphilis's dangers. One interesting offshoot of this latter effort was the VD Educational Record, a project by which Arkansas health officials commissioned artists and musicians like Allan Lomax to compose venereally themed songs bearing titles such as "That Ignorant, Ignorant Cowboy."[5] As a statistical table published in a 1951 edition of the *Arkansas Health Bulletin* made clear, the combined effect of these efforts was to substantially reduce the state's venereal burden.[6]

The Hot Springs VD clinic was integral to Arkansas's success in this matter. Though little is known about its day-to-day operations, the PHS clinic continued to operate in the period following Oliver C. Wenger's 1936 departure. In spite of the state's burgeoning antivenereal infrastructure, throughout the 1930s and 1940s those counties that lacked "complete" diagnostic and treatment facilities referred their venereally afflicted cases to the federal government's "model clinic." Rechristened the Hot Springs Medical Center, Wenger's establishment was transformed into a full-fledged research site by the clinic's medical doctors, whose experiments with penicillin and other advanced therapies earned it a designation as a "rapid treatment center."[7] After developing a method of treating venereal disease that required not months and years but *days* of medical care, the Hot Springs VD clinic quickly became the preferred source of antivenereal therapy among the state's health authorities, who increasingly concentrated their efforts on case finding.[8] As one public health worker put it, "If most or all infected cases can be sent to the United States Public Health Service Medical Center[,] . . . we believe venereal disease can be *stamped out*."[9]

Although Hot Springs played an important role in reducing Arkansas's venereal burden, in the years following Wenger's departure the city's medical center became an increasingly *insignificant* component of the nation's broader experience with syphilis.[10] To be sure, syphilis's relationship with Hot Springs did not simply disappear overnight, as throughout the late 1940s and 1950s, those who worked at the city's medical center conducted research on penicillin's antivenereal capabilities, enrolling the clinic's patients in therapeutic trials that resulted in publications bearing titles like "Treatment of Neurosyphilis at Hot Springs," "Electrocardiographic Changes in Secondary Syphilis," and "Penicillin-Resistant Gonorrhea versus Nonspecific Urethritis."[11] Yet with both the spread of penicillin and the growth of the nation's antivenereal clinical infrastructure, by the postwar period the cure of syphilis and gonorrhea had become a relatively easy, inexpensive, and quick affair, one that ultimately spelled the demise of Hot Springs as the medical destination for American syphilitics.[12]

With this, the city's privately practicing physicians lost their status as America's premier venereological experts. No longer valued for their skills in combating syphilis, from the mid-1930s onward, local doctors began applying the curative skills they had acquired through encounters with VD patients toward the cure of several other diseases commonly seen at the resort. Among these were arthritis, rheumatism, and poliomyelitis—all of which were said to yield to the same drugless, hydrotherapeutic regimen that syphilis did.[13] Much as was the case in earlier eras, when doctors argued for the benefits of what was now termed "pool therapy," they positioned Hot Springs as a place where patients entered a "different environment," one "away from business and other worries which would be present at home."[14] In response to skeptics who rejected the claim that the city's waters possessed unique healing properties, resident physicians drew attention to their highly radioactive nature, pointing out that the springs' radium emanations produced a "definite rise in body temperature" and the elimination of "waste material" through the skin, lungs, and kidneys.[15] Finally, in keeping with the holistic currents of interwar medicine, they contrasted their own "flexible" methods with the one-size-fits-all approach of most family physicians. "No two cases of arthritis are alike," one doctor observed, adding that the advantage of Hot Springs–based treatment owed to the fact that doctors here adapted regimens to "individual needs."[16]

Techniques such as these helped preserve Hot Springs' status as a prominent American health resort. As one local doctor noted, during the mid-1930s, "a large percentage" of the health seekers who traveled to the city were "now suffering from arthritis or chronic rheumatic disorders. Many of these are completely relieved," he observed, adding that "it is surprising at times to see the rapidity with which these cases improve, to note the reduction in the swelling of the joints, and the decrease in the stiffness and soreness in the muscles and ligaments. The relief from pain is often striking."[17] During the early 1940s, resident practitioners predicted that military conflict would increase the volume of medical tourist traffic within the city, especially as "the diseases which may be benefited by health resort therapy are definitely on the increase."[18] Interestingly, however, syphilitics were not among those listed as benefiting from a trip to Hot Springs. By the end of the Second World War, the phenomenon of venereal health seeking had come to an end.[19]

Interestingly, Hot Springs' fate was similar to that of other American health resorts in the postwar period. Productive of far more than penicillin, mid-twentieth century medical science witnessed the dawning of an era of "wonder drugs," as new medical technologies like antihistamines, corticosteroids, and antidepressants brought the country every closer to fulfilling its "a pill for every ill" mantra.[20] As a result of the availability of these novel "magic bullets," a preexisting regime of therapeutic practice rooted in the concept of "land health" fell by the wayside, bringing down with it the medical tourism industry that had sustained places as far flung as Denver, Tucson, and Saranac Lake throughout the late nineteenth and early twentieth centuries.[21] In keeping with these trends, public demand for Hot Springs' therapeutic services declined steadily throughout the late 1940s and early 1950s, as the city's private bathing establishments gradually went out of business and the federal government's free bathhouse closed its doors.[22]

In addition to being impacted by the federal government's stepped-up antivenereal efforts and the postwar period's therapeutic revolution, Hot Springs also felt the effect of shifting attitudes toward syphilis and gonorrhea within the United States. Upon assuming the directorship of the Hot Springs VD clinic, Oliver C. Wenger contended that while a "lack of facilities at home" and a popular belief in the healing qualities of its waters attracted the venereally afflicted to this southern city, also underwriting its identity as an asylum for Americans with syphilis was the fact that many VD patients "fear[ed] local ostracism" and so sought out a place where a "common bond" with others suffering from "the same affliction" would do "away with [the] embarrassment" they otherwise experienced.[23] Yet as Wenger's efforts illustrate, over the course of the interwar period the notion that America's venereal problems were the result of personal immorality and ignorance gradually gave way to a more humane, less stigmatized understanding of syphilis and gonorrhea. Partially as a result of its experiences in Hot Springs, by the 1940s the PHS had come to regard these maladies as the domain of medicine rather than morality, and as a result, the "ostracism" and "embarrassment" that had previously accompanied syphilis's contraction lost their status as the disease's most prominent symptoms.[24] And, as Wenger's remarks suggest, with the decline of the venereal stigma came the decline of the Hot Springs as a destination for syphilitics.[25]

As this account of the city's postwar development reminds us, Hot Springs' relationship to syphilis was a product of historical phenomena, of values and attitudes specific to time and place. Born of a set of beliefs native to late nineteenth- and early twentieth-century American culture, this southern city's venereal identity flowed from a medical mentality characterized by two lines of thought: the assumption that syphilis represented "the wages of sin" and the notion that health was a product of place and environment. In an era in which expanded clinic facilities and new "wonder drugs" like penicillin helped clear away the "hush-hush attitude" toward syphilis, such a mentality increasingly became a thing of the past, as did Hot Springs as the place for treatment of syphilis.[26]

Of course, the ties binding sexually transmitted illness to sexual immorality did not remain disconnected for long. With the coming of the AIDS crisis in the early 1980s, familiar arguments about the disease-inducing consequences of "sinful behavior" returned with a vengeance, as social, cultural, and political authorities constructed an etiological chain linking homosexuality, prostitution, drug use, and other deviant behaviors to the contraction of HIV. One outgrowth of these stigmatizing sentiments was the proposal to establish AIDS detention centers, where those infected with the virus would be quarantined and isolated from the "general public." Though lacking legislative support, calls to limit the geographical mobility of HIV-positive persons did exert a notable impact on American foreign policy: in 1987, the federal government introduced a ban on the entrance of HIV-positive immigrants into the country. Though repealed in 2010, the attitudes that informed this policy remain alive in many Western countries— most notably, the United Kingdom, where reactionary right-wing media outlets (especially the tabloid press) have positioned public health approaches aimed at ensuring universal access to antiretroviral therapies as a threat to national survival. With headlines such as "AIDS Epidemic Feared as Thousands of African Victims Pour into the UK" and "Migrants with AIDS Flood NHS," these publications stoke hysterical, unfounded fears of "AIDS tourists" draining the country's health care resources and leaving an immense trail of new HIV cases in their wake.[27] Though these sorts of claims are quickly rebutted by British medical professionals and governmental officials, they nevertheless speak to long-standing associations between sexually transmitted illness and health seeking behavior in the public mind.[28]

The focus of these discussions, however, stands in marked contrast to that of the early twentieth century. On account of AIDS' politicization as a national security concern, much of the debate today revolves around assessments of the risk HIV poses to travelers in certain parts of the world (specifically, countries in the global South). There are no conversations about particular locations that might be beneficial to people living with HIV and AIDS; rather the twenty-first century preoccupation is with how tourists can safeguard against the contraction of the virus and (as widespread fears of "AIDS tourists" indicate) with how the geographical mobility of those infected can be limited so as to prevent its spread. While not entirely new, these concerns underscore the uniquely exclusionary, nationalistic, and racialized geographical imaginary of many Western societies in the contemporary moment. As the history of Hot Springs shows, however, this perspective has not gone unchallenged. There have been other, perhaps more productive ways of configuring the relationship between sexually transmitted illness and health tourism.

How might the history of Hot Springs be of service to recent developments such as these? While it is difficult to extract particular "lessons" from its history, Hot Springs nevertheless presents an opportunity to move discussions about the twenty-first-century struggle against sexually transmitted infections forward. First and foremost, what the history of Hot Springs demonstrates is that stigma is not binding. Though limiting their therapeutic options, it did not deter people with VD from seeking out means of regaining health—either physically or mentally. And while discourses about the wages of sin fostered discriminatory behavior toward the infected, they were not completely determinative of syphilitics' illness experiences. Within the relatively destigmatized environment that was Hot Springs, patients often found ways not only to relieve mental and physical discomfort but also to forge meaningful human relationships and of developing a sense of belonging and purpose—all in spite of their ostracized status. Though their lives were far from ideal, the evidence from Hot Springs suggests that internalized feelings of shame and guilt did not exercise as much control over the thoughts and actions of people with VD as is commonly thought. From this, we can conclude that the best disease-control policies are those that acknowledge the humanity of the infected and afford opportunities for geographical mobility, peer support, and community building.

The second key insight Hot Springs yields has to do with the relationship between health outcomes and economic realities. For all of the emphasis that has been placed on the stigma and shame that pervade modern conceptions of sexually transmitted diseases, the concerns uppermost in the minds of the infected have often had more to do with money than morality. In the late nineteenth- and early twentieth-century United States, what complicated syphilitics' attempts to regain health was not simply prejudice or feelings of guilt but the immense financial complications of venereal illness—which often led to unemployment, loss of housing, and the depletion of personal savings due to costly medical treatments. Unable to support themselves, many of those who traveled to Hot Springs either returned home before completing their required courses of treatment or died in the city on account of pauperism. When in the 1930s the federal government began devoting its financial resources not only to free treatment but also to the promotion of patients' general well-being (such as the need for shelter, food, and basic medical care), the situation for many of the city's health seekers improved markedly. As its history thus demonstrates, solutions to the problems of sexually transmitted diseases that rely on market-based instruments are bound to fail; only with robust public sector investments in the health of the sick can societies begin to counteract and reverse the damages wrought by these maladies.

While the broad-based, environmental style of disease control that took shape in Hot Springs during the 1930s might be regarded as a model for contemporary campaigns to help people with HIV/AIDS, the city's history should also be read as a cautionary tale. As the existence of Camp Garraday illustrates, Hot Springs routinely set aside its most generous health care provisions for white males. As doctors formulated their first system of antivenereal praxis in the late nineteenth century, they offered rest cure to white patients while simultaneously contending that black syphilitics did not suffer from the psychological disturbances this regimen aimed to alleviate. On top of this, white healers contributed to existing patterns of racial discrimination within the city, excluding black doctors from the local association of medical professionals and subjecting black patients to regular doses of humiliation and disrespect. Sympathizing with white racial sensibilities, the PHS allowed Jim Crow to flourish within the city, even as officials such as Oliver Wenger rejected the idea that "immorality" explained blacks' higher rates of syphilis. Whereas white health seekers' emotional and economic difficulties were both validated and somewhat alleviated, this was much less the case for black visitors to the springs. The results of policies and practices such as these were predictable: their health care needs generally neglected, therapeutic outcomes for black patients were consistently worse than those of their white counterparts. Thus, although certain aspects of the city's response to syphilis might be deemed admirable, attempts to apply the "Hot Springs method" to the contemporary world must take heed: failure to do so in a racially equitable fashion will only exacerbate existing health inequalities.

Hot Springs' history as a hub for the treatment of syphilis can also be used to chart a way forward in VD historiography. Shifting attention to questions of medical practice is a fruitful way to examine the relationship between ideology and materiality—between social constructions of disease and bodily experience, therapeutic behavior, and clinical responses. As this study has shown, more than a mere ideological prop, throughout the late nineteenth and early twentieth centuries, syphilis was also a medical condition, one whose definition, diagnosis, and treatment bore the traces of an entire civilization's norms and values. Much important work remains to be done on this topic. In what other ways did the intermingling of "sin" and "science" produce novel therapeutic engagements with VD? To what extent did the racial, gendered, and class-based differences in health care outcomes seen in Hot Springs reproduce themselves in other contexts? And in what other ways have professional concerns shaped doctors' attempts to define, diagnose, and cure these conditions? Absent an engagement with matters pertaining to medical practice, an important part of the historical narrative will remain unwritten, and our knowledge of social responses to these conditions incomplete.

Subsequent research would also do well to highlight the salience of place. The systems of diagnosis and therapy that emerged in Hot Springs over the course of its history were the product of more general developments within the city. Shaped more by local institutions and actors than by national authorities or elite interests, the city's response to syphilis expressed the practical concerns, ideological attachments, physical needs, and personal aims of its inhabitants—be they visiting patients, resort healers, or permanent residents. While much of the extant scholarship on the era's "venereal peril" presents the federal government (especially the military and the PHS) as the key players in the fight against syphilis and gonorrhea, the evidence from Hot Springs points toward the opposite conclusion—that is, that the state's deliberations and decisions were *reactions* to those made by a variety of nonstate actors. Inserting these overlooked individuals into the historical narrative leads to a fundamentally new understanding of syphilis's meaning during a critical period in American history, to a radically different understanding of society's response to this disease, and to a much broader awareness of syphilis's significance in the context of contemporary medical developments. Thus, what the story of Hot Springs affords is not only a new narrative of the United States' venereal past but also a new perspective on the character and development of American medicine and public health in the five decades separating the triumph of germ theory and the dawning of the antibiotic era.

Of course, Hot Springs is but one stitch in the broader fabric that is the history of the United States' clinical encounter with sexually transmitted illnesses. In order to completely understand their embodied, corporeal, and material dimensions, in addition to the significance of local factors in shaping responses to them, the questions and themes brought to light here will need to be addressed in contexts outside of Hot Springs. Understanding them in all of their richness and complexity is critical to effectively solving the myriad problems presented by sexually transmitted infections; with this understanding lies the key to finally remedying the untold personal and collective damage that syphilis, gonorrhea, and HIV/AIDS have wrought upon our bodies, our minds, our societies, and our world.

Introduction

1. This letter comes from an online collection entitled "Taking the Waters: Nineteenth Century Medicinal Springs of Virginia," assembled by the University of Virginia's Claude Moore Health Sciences Library. For a full copy, see www.hsl.virginia.edu/historical /exhibits/springs/hot/banks.cfm.

2. D. H. Beckwith, "Public Health," in *Proceedings of the Thirty-Fourth Annual Session of the Homeopathic Medical Society of the State of Ohio* (Columbus: Spahr and Glenn, 1898), 76.

3. T. M. Baird, "Lesions of the Penis Simulating the Initial Lesions of Syphilis," *Journal of Materia Medica* 33:12 (1895): 191–92.

4. "Hot Springs and Syphilis," *Memphis Journal of the Medical Sciences* 3 (February 1892): 379.

5. See Loyd Thompson, *Syphilis* (Philadelphia: Lea and Febiger, 1920), 212. Numerous commentators spoke of Hot Springs in these terms over the course of the late nineteenth and early twentieth centuries. For other specific examples, see "Editorial: Syphilis of the Nervous System," *Hot Springs Medical Journal* 3:2 (1894): 51; Augustus Ravogli, "The Thermomineral Cure in the Treatment of Syphilis," *Medical Era* 6:8 (1897): 276; and Bukk G. Carleton, *A Treatise on Urological and Venereal Diseases* (New York: Bukk G. Carleton, 1905), 741.

6. Albert J. Whitworth and John M. Byrd, *The Hot Springs Specialist* (Memphis: B. C. Toof, 1913), 164.

7. Oliver C. Wenger, "Results of a Study and Investigation of Venereal Disease at the United States Public Health Service Clinic at Hot Springs, Arkansas," Oliver C. Wenger Papers, University of Arkansas for Medical Sciences Archives.

8. The term "medical tourism," it should be pointed out, is a problematic one. Among other concerns, scholars have drawn attention to the way it presents health travel as "a form of leisure or frivolity" (Beth Kangas, "Complicating Common Ideas about Medical Tourism: Gender, Class, and Globality in Yemenis' International Medical Travel," *Signs* 36:2 [2011]: 328).

9. Heather Hause, "Fountains of Youth: Medical Tourism in Green Cove Springs, Florida, 1845–1900," *Journal of Tourism History* 8:3 (2016): 239–59.

10. Conevery Bolton Valencius, *The Health of the Country: How American Settlers Understood Themselves and Their Land* (New York: Basic Books, 2002), 81.

11. Gregg Mitman, "In Search of Health: Landscape and Disease in American Environmental History," *Environmental History* 10:2 (2005): 184–210.

12. See also Katherine Ott, *Fevered Lives: Tuberculosis in American Culture since 1870* (Cambridge, MA: Harvard University Press, 1996).

13. Jeanne Abrams, "On the Road Again: Consumptives Traveling for Health in the American West, 1840–1925," *Great Plains Quarterly* 30:4 (2010): 271–85.

14. For more on "chasing the cure," see Sheila M. Rothman, *Living in the Shadow of Death: Tuberculosis and the Social Experience of Illness in the United States* (New York: Basic Books, 1994); Gregg Mitman, *Breathing Space: How Allergies Shape our Lives and Landscapes* (New Haven, CT: Yale University Press, 2007); and Joan M. Jensen, "Silver City Health Tourism in the Early Twentieth Century: A Case Study," *New Mexico Historical Review* 84:3 (2009): 321–61.

15. See Jane B. Donegan, *"Hydropathic Highway to Health": Women and Water-Cure in Antebellum America* (New York: Greenwood Press, 1986); and Susan E. Cayleff, *Wash and Be Healed: The Water-Cure Movement and Women's Health* (Philadelphia: Temple University Press, 1987).

16. See David Rosner, ed., *Hives of Sickness: Public Health and Epidemics in New York City* (New Brunswick, NJ: Rutgers University Press, 1995); Nancy Tomes, *The Gospel of Germs: Men, Women, and the Microbe in American Life* (Cambridge, MA: Harvard University Press, 1998); and Martin V. Melosi, *The Sanitary City: Environmental Services in Urban America from Colonial Times to the Present* (Pittsburgh: University of Pittsburgh Press, 2008).

17. Charles Rosenberg, "Pathologies of Progress: The Idea of Civilization as Risk," *Bulletin of the History of Medicine* 72:4 (1998): 714–30.

18. For a good overview of this subject, see Mitman, "In Search of Health." For additional studies, see W. Douglas McCombs, "Therapeutic Rusticity: Antimodernism, Health, and the Wilderness Vacation," *New York History* 76:4 (1995): 415–27; James C. Whorton, *Nature Cures: The History of Alternative Medicine in America* (New York: Oxford University Press, 2002); Conevery Bolton Valencius, "Gender and the Economy of Health on the Santa Fe Trail," *Osiris*, 2nd ser., 19 (2004): 79–92; Linda Nash, *Inescapable Ecologies: A History of Environment, Disease, and Knowledge* (Berkeley: University of California Press, 2006); and Emily K. Abel, *Tuberculosis and the Politics of Exclusion: A History of Public Health and Migration to Los Angeles* (New Brunswick, NJ: Rutgers University Press, 2007).

19. Frederick L. Hoffman, *A Plan for a More Effective Federal and State Health Administration* (Newark, NJ: Prudential Press, 1919), 80.

20. James J. Walsh, "The Inventor of Fresh Air," *Independent*, December 6, 1915, 405.

21. George B. Spencer, "Making People Healthwise," *New Outlook*, January 24, 1914, 222.

22. John V. Shoemaker, "The Advantages of the Pinellas Peninsula as a Resort and as a Home," *Medical Bulletin* 18:8 (1896): 281; "Water Gap Sanitarium," *Hall's Journal of Health* 40:6 (1893): 146.

23. "The Camp Cure," *Annals of Hygiene* 3:8 (1888): 310.

24. Ravogli, "The Thermomineral Cure in the Treatment of Syphilis," 276.

25. William Thomas Corlett, "Notes on the Treatment of Syphilis—Its Evolution and Present Status," in *Transactions of the Forty-Sixth Annual Meeting of the Ohio Medical Association* (Toledo, OH: Blade Printing and Paper Company, 1891), 90; G. Frank Lydston, *The Surgical Diseases of the Genito-Urinary Tract* (Philadelphia: F. A. Davis Company,

1904), 510; and Frederick R. Sturgis, "Indirect Methods of Treatment," *Medical Council* 14:4 (1909): 120.

26. J. B. McGee, "Syphilis," *Cleveland Medical Journal* 6:10 (1907): 437.

27. Edward L. Keyes and Charles H. Chetwood, *Venereal Diseases: Their Complications and Sequelae* (New York: William Wood and Company, 1900), 227. See also Ramon Guiteras, "The Treatment of Syphilis," *Journal of Cutaneous and Genito-Urinary Diseases* 16:4 (1898): 241.

28. Ravogli, "The Thermomineral Cure in the Treatment of Syphilis," 280. See also Alfred Lee Loomis and William Gilman Thompson, eds., *A System of Practical Medicine*, vol. 3 (New York: Lea Brothers, 1898), 250.

29. Albert H. Buck, ed., *Reference Handbook of the Medical Sciences*, vol. 4 (New York: William Wood and Company, 1902), 748.

30. William A. Mowry, "The Importance of a Specific Diet in General Practice," *Medical Times* 45:3 (1917): 64. See also Samuel G. Dabney, "Syphilitic Pharyngitis, Report of Two Cases," *American Journal Dermatology and Genito-Urinary Diseases* 18:5 (1914): 248–49; "Equal to Any European Spa," *Medical Standard* 40:5 (1917): 224; and Milton Goldsmith, "A Case of Hepatic Syphilis," *New York Medical Journal*, December 10, 1910, 1183–84.

31. "Proceedings of College of Physicians and Surgeons," *Medical Advance*, February 18, 1884, 669. A colleague noted that "we find that we are called upon to treat our patients for mercurialization more often than for latent syphilis" (John A. Lenfestey, "Infantile Syphilis," *Clinique* 28:11 [1907]: 657).

32. Sprague Carlton, "Salvarsan—Indications for and Methods of Use," *Journal of the American Institute of Homeopathy* 4:5 (1911–12): 539; John J. Moren, "Brown-Sequard Paralysis," *Louisville Monthly Journal of Medicine and Surgery* 17:3 (1910): 79.

33. John Kent Sanders, "Balneology: Facts and Fads of Baths and Bathing," *Medical Century: A Journal of Homeopathic Medicine and Surgery* 6:6 (1898): 177.

34. Lewis R. Morris, "The Therapeutic Action of Hot Sulpho-Saline Waters, with Some Personal Observations Made at Glenwood Hot Springs," *International Record of Medicine and General Practice*, September 28, 1895, 394.

35. Winslow Anderson, *Mineral Springs and Health Resorts of California* (San Francisco: Bancroft Company, 1890), 263.

36. Anderson, *Mineral Springs and Health Resorts of California*, 157.

37. Anderson, *Mineral Springs and Health Resorts of California*, 90.

38. G. M. Phillips, "In the Matter of Syphilis, Treatment of the Individual Is Scarcely Second in Importance to Treatment of the Disease," *Medical Mirror* 15:11 (1904): 374.

39. Phillips, "In the Matter of Syphilis, Treatment of the Individual Is Scarcely Second in Importance to Treatment of the Disease," 375.

40. Ravogli, "The Thermomineral Cure in the Treatment of Syphilis," 276.

41. Robert W. Taylor, *The Pathology and Treatment of Venereal Diseases* (Philadelphia: Lea Brothers, 1895), 908; Corlett, "Notes on the Treatment of Syphilis," 91.

42. "Influence of the Hot Springs of Arkansas on Syphilis," *Journal of Cutaneous and Genito-Urinary Diseases* 8:2 (1890): 66.

43. Lydston, *The Surgical Diseases of the Genito-Urinary Tract*, 510.

44. L. E. Russell, "Hot Springs, Arkansas," *Eclectic Medical Journal* 57:4 (1897): 207.

45. For examples of this scholarship, see Thomas A. Chambers, *Drinking the Waters: Creating an American Leisure Class at Nineteenth-Century Mineral Springs* (Washington,

DC: Smithsonian Institution Press, 2003); and Susan Barton, *Healthy Living in the Alps: The Origins of Winter Tourism in Switzerland, 1860–1914* (New York: Palgrave Macmillan, 2008).

46. For this, see especially Abel, *Tuberculosis and the Politics of Exclusion*.

47. Mitman, *Breathing Space*.

48. Mitman, *Breathing Space*, 104.

49. Meghan Crnic and Cynthia Connolly, "'They Can't Help Getting Well Here'": Seaside Hospitals for Children in the United States, 1872–1917," *Journal of the History of Childhood and Youth* 2:2 (2009): 220–33.

50. Walter D. Bierbach, "Venereal Disease and Prostitution," *Boston Medical and Surgical Journal* 172:6 (1915): 205.

51. Abraham L. Wolbarst, "The Venereal Diseases: A Menace to the National Welfare," *Medical Review* 62:10 (1910): 327–80; L. Duncan Bulkley, *Syphilis in the Innocent* (New York: Bailey and Forchild, 1894), 112.

52. Charles Greene Cumstom, "What Effective Measures Are There for the Prevention of the Spread of Syphilis and the Increase of Prostitution?" in *Transactions of the Section on Preventive and Industrial Medicine and Public Health of the American Medical Association* (Chicago: American Medical Association, 1906), 142.

53. George P. Dale, "Moral Prophylaxis," *American Journal of Nursing* 11 (July 1910): 609; Edward L. Keyes, *Syphilis: A Treatise for Practitioners* (New York: D. Appleton, 1908), 1; L. Duncan Bulkley, "Plain Truths about Syphilis," *Indiana Medical Journal* 26:3 (1907): 103.

54. G. Frank Lydston, *The Diseases of Society: The Vice and Crime Problem* (Philadelphia: Lippincott, 1908), 311; George M. Gould, *Borderland Studies*, vol. 2 (Philadelphia: Blakiston's Son, 1908), 103. For more estimates, see G. Shearman Peterkin, "A System of Venereal Prophylaxis That is Producing Results," *American Medicine* 10:8 (1906): 328. A colleague named John Cunningham declared that "it is a fact worthy of consideration that every year in this country 770,000 males reach the age of maturity. It may be affirmed that under existing conditions at least 60 percent, or over 450,000 of these young men will sometime during life become infected with venereal disease, if the experience of the past is to be accepted as a criterion of the future" ("The Importance of Venereal Disease," *New England Journal of Medicine* 168:3 [1913]: 77–78).

55. A number of turn-of-the-century books and pamphlets made use of this phrase; see in particular, Henry C. McHatton, *The Venereal Peril: Address to the Young Men of the Young Men's Christian Association* (Macon, GA: Smith and Watson, 1907); F. C. Valentine, *The Boy's Venereal Peril* (Chicago: American Medical Association, 1903); and William L. Holt and William J. Robinson, *The Venereal Peril: A Popular Treatise on Venereal Diseases* (New York: Altrurians, 1909). See also Charles Greene Cumstom, "What Effective Measures Are There for the Prevention of the Spread of Syphilis and the Increase of Prostitution?" in *Transactions of the Section on Preventive and Industrial Medicine and Public Health of the American Medical Association*, 142; Wolbarst, "The Venereal Diseases"; and Bulkley, *Syphilis in the Innocent*, 112.

56. "The Social Evil and the Report of the Committee of Fifteen," *Medical News*, April 19, 1902, 754.

57. Katie Johnson, "Damaged Goods: Sex Hysteria and the Prostitute Fatale," *Theatre Survey* 44:1 (2003): 43–68.

58. Helen Keller, "I Must Speak: A Plea to the American Woman," *Ladies' Home Journal* 26:2 (1909): 2.

59. William Lawrence, *Venereal Diseases in the Army, Navy, and Community* (New York: American Social Hygiene Association, 1918), 8.

60. Lawrence, *Venereal Diseases in the Army, Navy, and Community*, 1.

61. For a complete account of these discoveries, see J. D. Oriel, *The Scars of Venus: A History of Venereology* (Berlin: Springer, 1994). See also Karen J. Taylor, "Venereal Disease in Nineteenth-Century Children," *Journal of Psychohistory* 12:4 (1985): 431–63.

62. For information on one early figure in American venereology, see "Bumstead, Freeman J." in Howard A. Kelly and Walter L. Burrage, eds., *American Medical Biographies* (Baltimore, MD: Norman Remington Company, 1920), 171.

63. Leon L. Solomon, "Prevention and Control of Venereal Diseases," *Dental Summary* 39:12 (1919): 953.

64. Also known as "syphilitic myelopathy," tabes dorsalis is a condition characterized by the progressive degeneration of the nerves and nervous system and often leads to loss of coordination, dementia, and visual impairment. Along with insanity—most often diagnosed by turn-of-the-century doctors as a condition labeled "general paresis of the insane"—this was one of the most common manifestations of late-stage syphilis. For an incisive study of the medical profession's shifting understanding of these conditions, see Gayle Davis, *"The Cruel Madness of Love:" Sex, Psychiatry, and Syphilis in Scotland, 1880–1930* (Amsterdam: Rodopi, 2008).

65. Wolbarst, "The Venereal Diseases," 373.

66. Solomon, "Prevention and Control of Venereal Diseases," 953.

67. Whereas medical authorities dubbed tuberculosis the "white plague," syphilis was said to be the "red plague." See in particular, "Report of the Red Plague Committee," *Transactions of the Commonwealth Club of California* 8:7 (1913): 340.

68. The term "venereal peril" was a staple of turn-of-the-century discourse around syphilis and gonorrhea. For a particularly good example, see Holt and Robinson, *The Venereal Peril*.

69. Bulkley, *Syphilis in the Innocent*, 112.

70. "Syphilis—How Shall We Stop Its Alarming Spread," *Gaillard's Medical Journal* 70:7 (1899): 404.

71. "Syphilis," 404.

72. Curtis R. Day, "Venereal Infections, with Reference to Criminal, Mental, and Nervous Disturbances," *Journal of the Oklahoma Medical Association* 5:4 (1912): 143.

73. Day, "Venereal Infections," 143.

74. Charles Francis White and William Herbert Brown, *An Atlas of the Primary and Cutaneous Lesions of Acquired Syphilis* (New York: William Wood, 1920), 3.

75. Bulkley, *Syphilis in the Innocent*, 112; W. J. Craddock, "Hereditary Transmission," *Medical Times and Register* 37:8 (1899): 259.

76. J. Ewing Myers, "The Problem of the Social Evil Considered in the Social and Medical Aspects and in Its Relation to the Problem of Race Betterment," *Medical Record*, December 27, 1913, 234.

77. "Etiology of General Paralysis of the Insane," *Journal of the American Medical Association* 34:2 (1900): 1635.

78. Ferd C. Valentine, "Educational Limitation of Venereal Diseases," *Medical Record,* November 8, 1902, 74.

79. W. L. Allen, "The Social Evil—Should It Be Regulated? Can It Be Exterminated?" *Journal of the American Medical Association* 28:11 (1897): 481.

80. "Second International Conference for the Prevention of Syphilis and Venereal Diseases," *Medical News,* September 20, 1902, 572.

81. Ludwig Weiss, "Venereal Prophylaxis That Is Feasible," *Journal of the American Medical Association* 40:1 (1903): 232.

82. Weiss, "Venereal Prophylaxis That Is Feasible," 232.

83. Weiss, "Venereal Prophylaxis That Is Feasible," 232. As Mary Spongberg explains, it was during the nineteenth century that the pathologization of the prostitute's body reached its apogee (*Feminizing Venereal Disease: The Body of the Prostitute in Nineteenth-Century Medical Discourse* [New York: New York University Press, 1998]).

84. G. A. Pudor, "Prevention of Venereal Diseases," *Journal of Medicine and Science* 11:2 (1905): 38.

85. "New York County Medical Society," *Medical News,* March 23, 1901, 481.

86. Robert L. Griswold, "Sexual Cruelty and the Case for Divorce in Victorian America," *Signs: Journal of Women in Culture and Society* 11:3 (1986): 529–41; Steven Ruggles, "The Rise of Divorce and Separation in the United States, 1880–1990," *Demography* 34:4 (1997): 455–66.

87. See also Allan Brandt, *No Magic Bullet: A Social History of Venereal Disease in the United States since 1880* (New York: Oxford University Press, 1987).

88. For one example of this, see Douglas M. Peers, "Soldiers, Surgeons, and the Campaign to Combat Sexually-Transmitted Diseases in Colonial India," *Medical History* 42:2 (1998): 137–60.

89. For representative examples of this scholarship, see Kerrie Macpherson, "Health and Empire: Britain's National Campaign to Combat Venereal Diseases in Shanghai, Hong Kong, and Singapore," in *Sex, Sin, and Suffering: Venereal Disease and European Society since 1870,* ed. Roger Davidson and Lesley A. Hall (New York: Routledge, 2001), 173–90; Karen Jochelson, *The Colour of Disease: Syphilis and Racism in South Africa, 1880–1950* (New York: Palgrave Macmillan, 2001); Frank Proschan, "'Syphilis, Opiomania, and Pederasty': Colonial Constructions of Vietnamese (and French) Social Diseases," *Journal of the History of Sexuality* 11:4 (2002), 610–36; Ashwini Tambe, *Codes of Misconduct: Regulating Prostitution in Late Colonial Bombay* (Minneapolis: University of Minnesota Press, 2009); Erica Wald, *Vice in the Barracks: Medicine, the Military, and the Making of Colonial India, 1780–1868* (New York: Palgrave Macmillan, 2014); Saheed Aderinto, *When Sex Threatened the State: Illicit Sexuality, Nationalism, and Politics in Colonial Nigeria, 1900–1958* (Urbana: University of Illinois Press, 2015); and Daniel J. Walther, *Sex and Control: Venereal Disease, Colonial Physicians, and Indigenous Agency in German Colonialism, 1884–1914* (New York: Berghahn, 2015).

90. For a discussion of how British officials expanded the definition of prostitution in India, see Erica Wald, "From *Begums* and *Bibis* to Abandoned Females and Idle Women: Sexual Relationships, Venereal Disease, and the Redefinition of Prostitution in Early Nineteenth-Century India," *Indian Economic and Social History Review* 46:1 (2009): 5–25. For a general discussion of VD in British India, see Philippa Levine, *Prostitution, Race, and Politics: Policing Venereal Disease in the British Empire* (New York: Routledge, 2003).

91. For a particularly good discussion of how colonized women turned VD policies toward their own ends, see Sarah Hodges, "'Looting' the Lock Hospital in Colonial Madras during the Famine Years of the 1870s," *Social History of Medicine* 18:3 (2005): 379–98.

92. "Science and Alcohol," *National Advocate* 47:2 (1912): 20.

93. Edward L. Munson, *The Theory and Practice of Military Hygiene* (London: Bailliere, Tindall, and Box, 1902), 823.

94. William F. Snow and Wilbur A. Sawyer, "Venereal Disease Control in the Army," *Journal of the American Medical Association* 71:1 (1918): 456–57.

95. For an especially enlightened discussion of these fears, see Chad Heap, *Slumming: Sexual and Racial Encounters in American Nightlife, 1885–1940* (Chicago: University of Chicago Press, 2010).

96. For a discussion of this, see Marilyn Hegarty, *Victory Girls, Khaki-Wackies, and Patriotutes: The Regulation of Female Sexuality during World War Two* (New York: New York University Press, 2008). For more on the history of prostitution in the modern United States, see Mark T. Connelly, *The Response to Prostitution in the Progressive Era* (Chapel Hill: University of North Carolina Press, 1980); Ruth Rosen, *The Lost Sisterhood: Prostitution in America, 1900–1918* (Baltimore, MD: Johns Hopkins University Press, 1982); Brian Donovan, *White Slave Crusades: Race, Gender, and Anti-Vice Activism, 1887–1917* (Urbana: University of Illinois Press, 2006); Elizabeth Alice Clement, *Love for Sale: Courting, Treating, and Prostitution in New York City, 1900–1945* (Chapel Hill: University of North Carolina Press, 2006); and Mara L. Keire, *For Business and Pleasure: Red-Light Districts and the Regulation of Vice in the United States, 1890–1933* (Baltimore, MD: Johns Hopkins University Press, 2010).

97. Paul Lombardo, "A Child's Right to Be Well-Born: Venereal Disease and the Eugenic Marriage Laws, 1913–1935," *Perspectives in Biology and Medicine* 60:2 (2017): 211–32. See also Pippa Holloway, *Sexuality, Politics, and Social Control in Virginia, 1920–1945* (Chapel Hill: University of North Carolina Press, 2006).

98. For a recent analysis of VD reporting laws, see Amy L. Fairchild, Ronald Bayer, and James Colgrove, *Searching Eyes: Privacy, the State, and Disease Surveillance in America* (Berkeley: University of California Press, 2009). And for an account of VD and immigration inspections, see Amy L. Fairchild, *Science at the Borders: Immigrant Medical Inspection and the Shaping of the Modern Industrial Labor Force* (Baltimore, MD: Johns Hopkins University Press, 2003).

99. Alexandra M. Lord, "'Naturally Clean and Wholesome': Women, Sex Education, and the United States Public Health Service, 1928–1938," *Social History of Medicine* 17:3 (2004): 423–41.

100. Joshua Gamson, "Rubber Wars: Struggles over the Condom in the United States," *Journal of the History of Sexuality* 1:2 (1990): 262–82. See also Alexandra M. Lord, *Condom Nation: The US Government's Sex Education Campaign from World War I to the Internet* (Baltimore, MD: Johns Hopkins University Press, 2010).

101. Dale, "Moral Prophylaxis," 782.

102. James Jones, *Bad Blood: The Tuskegee Syphilis Experiment* (New York: Free Press, 1981), 106. See also Susan Reverby, *Examining Tuskegee: The Infamous Syphilis Study and its Legacy* (Chapel Hill: University of North Carolina Press, 2009).

103. For more on this, see Suzanne Poirier, *Chicago's War on Syphilis, 1937–40: The Times, the "Trib," and the Clap Doctor* (Urbana: University of Illinois Press, 1995).

104. Elizabeth Fee, "Sin v. Science: Venereal Disease in Baltimore in the Twentieth Century," *Journal of the History of Medicine and Allied Sciences* 43:2 (1988): 145.

105. Brandt, *No Magic Bullet*, 182.

106. Brandt, *No Magic Bullet*, 5, 31.

107. According to Brandt, the reason so many doctors, scientists, and medical officials saw syphilis as a sign of "moral decay" had to do with preexisting fears about a "family crisis." Believing that this venereal disease contributed the era's increasing divorce rate, its declining birth rate, the "growing tendency toward later marriages," and the growing number of women who "passed up domestic life altogether," medico-scientific authorities treated syphilis as one of the key causes of the breakup of the white, middle-class family—and by extension, as "an actual cause of the degeneration of the race" (*No Magic Bullet*, 7, 16).

108. For relevant examples, see Theodor Rosebury, *Microbes and Morals: The Strange Story of Venereal Disease* (New York: Viking, 1971); Jones, *Bad Blood*; Poirier, *Chicago's War on Syphilis*; Nancy K. Bristow, *Making Men Moral: Social Engineering during the Great War* (New York: New York University Press, 1996); Andrea Tone, *Devices and Desires: A History of Contraceptives in America* (New York: Hill and Wang, 2000); Hegarty, *Victory Girls, Khaki-Wackies, and Patriotutes*; John Parascandola, *Sex, Sin, and Science: A History of Syphilis in America* (Westport, CT: Praeger, 2008); Lynn Sacco, *Unspeakable: A History of Father-Daughter Incest in American History* (Baltimore, MD: Johns Hopkins University Press, 2009); and Reverby, *Examining Tuskegee.*

109. Brandt, *No Magic Bullet*, 23.

110. Kevin P. Sienna, *Venereal Disease, Hospitals, and the Urban Poor: London's "Foul Wards," 1600–1800* (Rochester, NY: University of Rochester Press, 2004), 16.

111. Antje Kampf, *Mapping out the Venereal Wilderness: Public Health and STD in New Zealand, 1920–80* (Piscataway, NJ: Transaction, 2007), 107, 3.

112. Roger Davidson, *Dangerous Liaisons: A Social History of Venereal Disease in Twentieth-Century Scotland* (Amsterdam: Rodopi, 2000), 64. Stressing this point, Klara Hribkova observes that even if early twentieth-century doctors had successfully abandoned the preconceptions of middle-class morality, VD would still have been a difficult problem. "No amount of funds could have possibly helped stamp VD out," she writes, "when the whole administrative and organizational structure of clinical medicine—the *techniques* such as record-keeping and follow-up—were not yet in place" ("Power, Subject, and Syphilis: Towards a Sociology of Venereal Disease in the United States, 1900–1950" [PhD diss., Simon Fraser University, 2004], 12).

113. Anne Hanley, *Medicine, Knowledge, and Venereal Diseases in England, 1886–1916* (New York: Palgrave MacMillan, 2017), 11. For another excellent study probing these connections, see Davis, *"The Cruel Madness of Love."*

114. Sienna, *Venereal Disease, Hospitals, and the Urban Poor*, 265.

115. One of the only historical analyses of syphilis to focus on the disease's chronic side is Laura J. McGough, *Gender, Sexuality, and Syphilis in Early Modern Venice: The Disease that Came to Stay* (Basingstoke, UK: Palgrave Macmillan, 2011).

116. Laura J. McGough and Katherine E. Bliss, "Sex and Disease from Syphilis to AIDS," in *A Global History of Sexuality: The Modern Era*, ed. Robert M. Buffington, Eithne Luibhéid, and Donna J. Guy (Malden, MA: Wiley-Blackwell, 2014), 114.

117. Sacco, *Unspeakable*, 117, 126.

118. Lynn Sacco, "Sanitized for Your Protection: Medical Discourse and the Denial of Incest in the United States, 1890–1940," *Journal of Women's History* 14:3 (2002): 90.

119. For attempts to do this within the context of early modern Europe, see Kevin Sienna, ed., *Sins of the Flesh: Responding to Sexual Disease in Early Modern Europe* (Toronto: Centre for Reformation and Renaissance Studies, 2005); and Cristian Berco, *From Body to Community: Venereal Disease and Society in Baroque Spain* (Toronto: University of Toronto Press, 2016).

120. Brandt, *No Magic Bullet*, 178.

121. Brandt, *No Magic Bullet*, 5.

122. Oliver C. Wenger, "The Need for Social Hygiene," Wenger Papers.

Chapter 1 · *The Emergence of Hot Springs as a Haven*

1. Information on Cowles's life comes courtesy of the Garland County Historical Society, Hot Springs, AR, repository of Cowles's papers. For the aforementioned descriptions of his illness, see the letters Cowles penned on April 29, 1906, May 8, 1906, May 27, 1906, and May 5, 1907.

2. Allan Brandt, *No Magic Bullet: A Social History of Venereal Disease in the United States since 1880* (New York: Oxford University Press, 1987), 5.

3. For relevant examples, see Theodor Rosebury, *Microbes and Morals: The Strange Story of Venereal Disease* (New York: Viking, 1971); Suzanne Poirier, *Chicago's War on Syphilis, 1937–40: The Times, the "Trib," and the Clap Doctor* (Urbana: University of Illinois Press, 1995); Nancy K. Bristow, *Making Men Moral: Social Engineering during the Great War* (New York: New York University Press, 1996); Marilyn Hegarty, *Victory Girls, Khaki-Wackies, and Patriotutes: The Regulation of Female Sexuality during World War Two* (New York: New York University Press, 2008); and John Parascandola, *Sex, Sin, and Science: A History of Syphilis in America* (Westport, CT: Praeger, 2008).

4. Explaining his rejection of this offer, Cowles wrote to his friend that "Amy has plenty of worry and it is an extra burden to have someone sick in the house."

5. "I appreciate your offer of $5.00 and it shows you are a true friend," Cowles wrote one of these friends on May 11, 1906. "My father is going to help me," he added in a later letter, dated June 20, 1907, noting that "I want some money of my own too."

6. For more on the city's early history and the role of the Hot Springs Reservation, see Janis Kent Percefull, *Ouachita Springs Region: A Curiosity of Nature* (Hot Springs, AR: Ouchita Springs Region Historical Research Center, 2007). For more on the geology of Hot Springs, see John C. Paige and Laura Soulliere Harrison, *Out of the Vapors: A Social and Architectural History of Bathhouse Row* (Washington, DC: National Park Service, 1988), 19–20.

7. R. M. Lackey, "The Hot Springs of Arkansas," *Chicago Medical Journal* 23:1 (1866): 9; A. J. Wright, "Some Account of the Hot Springs of Arkansas," *New Orleans Medical and Surgical Journal* (1860): 801. See also J. L. White, "The Hot Springs of Arkansas," *Chicago Medical Journal and Examiner* 36:3 (1878): 311.

8. J. K. Haywood, *Analyses of the Waters of the Hot Springs of Arkansas* (Washington, DC: Government Printing Office, 1912), 5.

9. For more on this, see Conevery Bolton Valencius, *The Health of the Country: How American Settlers Understood Themselves and Their Land* (New York: Basic Books, 2002).

10. Seale Harris, "Prevention of Malaria," *Journal of the American Medical Association* 53:2 (1909): 1162.

11. E. G. Epler, "The Climate and Mortality of Fort Smith, Arkansas," *Climatologist* 2:5 (1892): 303.

12. Conevery Bolton Valencius, "The Geography of Health and the Making of the American West: Arkansas and Missouri, 1800–1860," in *Medical Geography in Historical Perspective*, ed. Nicolaas A. Rupke (London: Wellcome Trust Center for the History of Medicine, 2000), 125.

13. Jerome Jansma, Harriet J. Jansma, and George Engelmann, "George Englemann in Arkansas Territory," *Arkansas Historical Quarterly* 50:3 (1991): 242–43.

14. W. J. Goulding, "Medical Topography of Central Arkansas: Being Observations on the Locality, Climate, and Diseases of the City of Little Rock and Vicinity, in the Year 1840," *Western Journal of Medicine and Surgery* 7 (May 1843): 324.

15. T. B. Mills and Company, *A History of the North-Western Editorial Excursion to Arkansas* (Little Rock, AR: T. B. Mills and Company, 1876), 371; "The Electric Springs Sanitarium," *Eclectic Medical Journal* 65:5 (1905): 292.

16. Randolph Brunson, "Address of Welcome to the Arkansas Medical Society during the Annual Meeting at Hot Springs," *Hot Springs Medical Journal* 10:5 (1901): 163. For a discussion of malaria's slow retreat from the American South, see Margaret Humphreys, *Malaria: Race, Poverty, and Public Health in the United States* (Baltimore, MD: Johns Hopkins University Press, 2001).

17. Frederick L. Wachenheim, *The Climatic Treatment of Children* (New York: Rebman Company, 1907), 158.

18. Charles Dake, "Hot Springs, Arkansas," *Medical Century*, November 15, 1894, 536.

19. T. B. Mills and Company, *A History of the North-Western Editorial Excursion to Arkansas*, 370.

20. *Arkansas: Statistics and Information Showing Its Agricultural and Mineral Resources* (Iron Mountain Route, 1903), 17; J. C. McMechan, "The Hot Springs of Arkansas," *Cincinnati Lancet and Clinic* 49:10 (1882): 131.

21. For some of the more popular guidebooks, see Charles Cutter, *The Hot Springs of Arkansas as They Are: A History and Guide* (Hot Springs, AR: Courier-Advertiser Printing House,1876); Algernon S. Garnett, *A Treatise on the Hot Springs of Arkansas* (St. Louis, MO: Von Beek, Barnard and Tinsley, 1874).

22. For evidence of this, see Edward L. Keyes, "Influence of the Hot Springs in Arkansas on Syphilis," *Journal of Cutaneous Diseases Including Syphilis* 8:2 (1890): 64; Eugene Carson Hay, "Modern Methods of Treating Syphilis," in *Transactions of the Mississippi Valley Medical Association* (Kansas City, MO: Burd and Fletcher, 1903), 278–79.

23. For one example of this, see the advertisement for "the Hot Springs Remedy" in *Out West: A Magazine of the Old Pacific and the New* 7 (March 1914): 170.

24. See, for example, Harry H. Myers, "Hot Springs, Arkansas, the World's Sanatorium and Pleasure Resort," *Journal of the Arkansas Medical Society* 8:11 (1911): 299.

25. Moses Foster Sweetser, *King's Handbook of the United States* (Buffalo, NY: Moses King Corporation, 1892), 63.

26. S. B. Houts, "Cases in Practice," *Medical World* 5:7 (1887): 248–52; Edward L. Keyes, *The Venereal Diseases, Including Stricture of the Male Urethra* (New York: William Wood and Company, 1880), 107–8.

27. E. R. Lewis, "The Hot Springs of Arkansaw," *Kansas City Medical Index-Lancet* 10:7 (1889): 249.

28. *Arkansas: Statistics and Information Showing Its Agricultural and Mineral Resources*, 20.

29. C. F. Ellis, "Eureka Springs, Arkansas," *Medical Century*, November 15, 1894, 535.

30. Speaking of the "unfortunate" showers that sometimes blanketed the city, this visitor opined that "the water which comes down from above seems to be trying to wash out all the beneficial effects which come from the waters of the hot springs below" ("A Health Resort," *Advance*, April 27, 1911, 519).

31. E. B. Stevens, "Hot Springs, Arkansas," in *Transactions of the Ohio Medical Society* 31 (Cincinnati, OH: A. H. Pounsford, 1875), 197. Noting that its boarding and bathing accommodations were "scarcely sufficient for one-hundred persons," a Chicago medical man who visited the city in 1866 claimed that many of Hot Springs' health seekers "partake of the character—physically, mentally, and morally—that so invariably pertains to the poor whites of the South (R. M. Lackey, "The Hot Springs of Arkansas," *Chicago Medical Journal* 23:1 [1866]: 9).

32. "Observations at Hot Springs, Arkansas," *Medical and Surgical Reporter*, January 29, 1881, 137–38.

33. J. L. Gebhart, "On the Therapy of the Waters of Hot Springs, Arkansas, and Their Relation to the Medical Profession at Large," *St. Louis Medical and Surgical Journal*, June 20, 1880, 634.

34. Robert Heriot, "Letter to the Editor," *Locomotive Engineers Journal* 25:10 (1891): 919.

35. For more on the city's luxurious accommodations, see Henry Durand, "Uncle Sam, M.D., and His Great Sanitarium," *American Monthly Review of Reviews* 16 (December 1897): 75–79; J. P. Dake, "Correspondence," *Medical Counselor* 8:18 (1884): 644–46.

36. Carolyn Thomas de la Peña, "Recharging at the Fordyce: Confronting the Machine and Nature in the Modern Bath," *Technology and Culture* 40:4 (1999): 754.

37. For a complete discussion of the Maurice Bathhouse, see Paige and Harrison, *Out of the Vapors*, 50–53.

38. "Hot Springs, Arkansas," *Medical Visitor* 20:4 (1904): 140; "Hot Springs, Arkansas, as a Health Resort," *Hot Springs Medical Journal* 3:6 (1894): 173; William H. Deaderick, "The Development of the Hot Springs of Arkansas as a Health Resort," *Medical Pickwick* 2:7 (1916): 265–66.

39. Kathryn Carpenter, "'Cesspools,' Springs, and Snaking Pipes," *Technology's Stories*, March 13, 2019, www.technologystories.org/cesspools-springs.

40. For more on this, see Kathryn Carpenter, "Access to Nature, Access to Health: The Government Free Bathhouse at Hot Springs National Park, 1877–1922," MA thesis, University of Missouri, 2019.

41. Hal C. Wyman, "A Surgical Pilgrimage to Arkansas," *Physician and Surgeon* 28:5 (1906): 207.

42. Carpenter, "'Cesspools,' Springs, and Snaking Pipes."

43. Heriot, "Letter to the Editor," 919. See also H. M. Rector, "Then and Now," *Hot Springs Medical Journal* 4:8 (1895): 225; Durand, "Uncle Sam, M.D., and His Great Sanitarium," 75–79.

44. "Hot Springs, Arkansas," 140; "Hot Springs, Arkansas, as a Health Resort," 173. For an interesting case of a neurasthenic doctor treated in Hot Springs, see Hans Froelich, "The New Era for Hot Springs," *Hot Springs Medical Journal* 3:2 (1894): 35–39.

45. "Syphilitic Paresis," *Eclectic Medical Journal* 50:11 (1890): 562.

46. Joseph Zeisler, "The Social Evil," *Year Book* (Chicago: Sunset Club, 1894), 218.

47. J. M. Keller, "The Hot Springs of Arkansas as a Health Resort," *St. Louis Medical and Surgical Journal* 37:2 (1879): 89.

48. Prince A. Morrow, "The Prophylaxis of Venereal Diseases," *Philadelphia Medical Journal*, April 6, 1901, 665.

49. Henry H. Morton, *Genitourinary Diseases and Syphilis* (St. Louis, MO: C. V. Mosby Company, 1918), 233; Reuben Peterson, "A Plea for Routine Wassermann Examinations for Obstetric and Gynecologic Patients in Hospital and General Practice," *American Journal of Syphilis* 1:1 (1917): 212.

50. Morrow, "The Prophylaxis of Venereal Diseases," 665.

51. "Syphilis," *California Medical and Surgical Reporter* 1:3 (1905): 283.

52. Arthur Shillitoe, "Syphilis in Women," in *The New System of Gynaecology*, ed. Thomas W. Eden and Cuthbert Lockyer, vol. 1 (London: Macmillan, 1917), 680.

53. John H. Stokes, *The Third Great Plague* (Philadelphia: W. B. Saunders, 1917), 120.

54. For an example of a woman with syphilis who was unable to travel to Hot Springs, see R. W. Taylor, "History of a Case of Syphilis Fourteen Years after the Onset of Cerebral Symptoms," *Journal of Cutaneous Diseases Including Syphilis* 8:3 (1890): 81–90.

55. For the details of this case, see "Koehler v. Koehler," *Southwestern Reporter* 209 (February 17, 1919): 283–85.

56. For a record of this case, see "Wilson v. Wilson," *Southwest Reporter* 134 (March 8–March 29, 1912): 963–67.

57. For the details of this case, see "Wade v. Wade," *Southwestern Reporter* 229 (May 11–June 1, 1921): 432.

58. For discussions of Grand's work, see Emma Liggins, "Writing against the 'Husband-Fiend': Syphilis and Male Sexual Vice in the New Woman Novel," *Women's Writing* 7:2 (2000): 175–95; Meegan Kennedy, "Syphilis and the Hysterical Female: The Limits of Realism in Sarah Grand's *The Heavenly Twins*," *Women's Writing* 11:2 (2004): 259–80; and William Driscoll, "The Metaphor of Syphilis in Grand's *Heavenly Twins*," *Nineteenth-Century Gender Studies* 5:1 (2009): 350–72.

59. For a discussion of this in the context of England, see Gail Savage, "'The Willful Communication of a Loathsome Disease': Marital Conflict and Venereal Disease in Victorian England," *Victorian Studies* 34:1 (1990): 35–54. For another study looking at the relationship between VD and the courts, see Victoria Bates, "'So Far as I Can Define without a Microscopical Examination': Venereal Disease Diagnosis in English Courts, 1850–1914," *Social History of Medicine* 26:1 (2012): 38–55.

60. For discussions of this, see Ann Taylor Allen, "Feminism, Venereal Diseases, and the State in Germany, 1890–1918," *Journal of the History of Sexuality* 4:1 (1993): 27–50, and Michael Worboys, "Unsexing Gonorrhoea: Bacteriologists, Gynaecologists, and Suffragists in Britain," *Social History of Medicine* 17:1 (2004): 41–59.

61. As one recent volume puts it, the prevailing belief at the time was that "when men spread syphilis, it was unfortunate; when women spread it, it was reprehensible" (W. F. Bynum, Anne Hardy, Stephen Jayca, Christopher Lawrence, and E. M. Tansey, *The Western Medical Tradition, 1800–2000* [New York: Cambridge University Press, 2006], 179).

62. For an analysis of how these antiprostitution drives played out in the US South, see Jamie Schmidt Wagman, "Women Reformers Respond during the Depression: Battling St. Louis's Disease and Immorality," *Journal of Urban History* 35:5 (2009): 698–719.

63. White, "The Hot Springs of Arkansas," 312.

64. "The Non-Institutional Treatment of Syphilis," *Journal of Physical Therapy* 1:12 (1905): 564.

65. Conevery Bolton Valencius, "Gender and the Economy of Health on the Santa Fe Trail," *Osiris*, 2nd ser., 19 (2004): 89. For a contemporary example, see James E. Dalen, "Medical Tourists: Incoming and Outgoing," *American Journal of Medicine* 132:1 (2019): 9–10.

66. For evidence of these religiously inflected understandings of syphilis, see E. A. King and F. B. Meyer, *Clean and Strong: A Book for Young Men* (Boston: United Society of Christian Endeavors, 1909), 112; and Alfred Fournier, *The Treatment and Prophylaxis of Syphilis* (New York: Rebman Company, 1907), 524.

67. "Editorial: The Moral Etiology of Syphilis," *Journal of Cutaneous Diseases Including Syphilis* 21:2 (1903): 57.

68. "Editorial: The Moral Etiology of Syphilis," 58.

69. As Cowles departed Ohio in 1907, a Toledo hospital's patient admission guidelines declared that "no contagious, chronic or incurable diseases, and no venereal disease consequent upon the immorality of the person shall be admitted for treatment" (*Annual Report of the Toledo Hospital for the Year Ending December 31st, 1907* [Toledo, OH: Board of Trustees, 1907], 58). Similar policies prevailed at major urban hospitals across the country. For more on this, see William S. Gottheil, "The Systematic Treatment of Syphilis," *Post-Graduate* 22:2 (1907): 126; John B. Roberts, "The Physician's Part in the War against Venereal Diseases," *International Clinics* 3:20 (1910): 244–52; and James Pedersen, "How Can Prophylaxis by Treatment in the Case of Venereal Diseases Be Obtained?" *New York Medical Journal*, April 6, 1907, 637–39.

70. J. L. Tracy, "The Attitude of the Medical Profession towards Prostitution," *Cincinnati Medical Journal* 4:6 (1889): 198. For others, the appropriate approach was not to callously deny treatment but instead to make them pay "far more" than other patients—the excessive doctors' fees levied "as a punishment for their evil ways." For evidence of this practice, see "Editorial," *Lancet*, September 1887, 350.

71. Indiana Board of Health, *Social Hygiene vs. The Sexual Plagues* (Indianapolis: Indiana Board of Health, 1910), 15.

72. Theodore Schroeder, *Freedom of the Press and "Obscene" Literature: Three Essays* (New York: Free Speech League, 1906): 25; Frank Wieland, "Treatment of Gonorrhea," *Medical Forum* 1:5 (1904): 198.

73. For an important study dealing with venereological training, see Anne R. Hanley, *Medicine, Knowledge, and Venereal Diseases in England, 1886–1916* (London: Palgrave Macmillan, 2017).

74. L. H. Van Buskirk, "The Laboratory and Venereal Diseases," *Ohio Public Health Journal* 9:7 (1918): 305.

75. F. L. Bott, "Gonorrhea, the Great Evil of the Day," *Medical World* 28:10 (1910): 423.

76. For evidence of mercury's unpopularity, see Isaac Newton Love, "Book Shelf," *Medical Mirror*, June 1, 1890, 307; D'Arcy Power and J. Keogh Murphy, eds., *A System of Syphilis*, vol. 2 (London: Oxford University Press, 1908), 261; Albert E. Carrier, "Syphilis, Its Management and Control," *Journal of the Michigan State Medical Society* 2:5 (1903): 190; Edward L. Keyes, "The Treatment of Syphilis in Its Different Stages," *Philadelphia Medical Times*, February 25, 1882, 337–44; and Edward L. Keyes and Charles H. Chetwood,

Venereal Diseases: Their Complications and Sequelae (New York: William Wood, 1900). For the European public's equally hostile reception of this unpopular compound, see Alfred Fournier, *The Treatment and Prophylaxis of Syphilis*, trans. C. F. Marshall (New York: Berman, 1907), 196.

77. Carrier, "Syphilis, Its Management and Control," 190; Fournier, *The Treatment and Prophylaxis of Syphilis*, 59; Robert W. Taylor, *The Pathology and Treatment of Venereal Diseases* (Philadelphia: Lea Brothers, 1895), 825.

78. Edward L. Keyes, *The Tonic Treatment of Syphilis* (New York: Appleton, 1896), 49. According to the French syphilographer Albert Fournier, little of the "contradictions and formidable opposition" that followed the use of mercury seemed to blot the iodides' reputation, though as he noted this drug too had its associated "disadvantages" and "dangers" (*The Treatment of Syphilis*, 180, 182–83). For evidence of physicians' positive evaluations of mercury and the iodides, see L. Duncan Bulkley, "On the Relative Value of Mercury and Iodine Compounds in the Treatment of Syphilis," *Journal of the American Medical Association* 15:22 (1890): 773–75; L. Duncan Bulkley, *Manual of Diseases of the Skin* (New York: G. P. Putnam and Sons, 1895), 132; Taylor, *The Pathology and Treatment of Venereal Diseases*, esp. 820–919; Keyes, *The Tonic Treatment of Syphilis*; Fournier, *The Treatment of Syphilis*, esp. 180–192; Augustus Ravogli, *Syphilis in Its Medical, Medico-Legal, and Sociological Aspects* (New York: Grafton Press, 1907), esp. 148, 218; Hermann G. Klotz, "What Can Treatment Do for the Prophylaxis of the Venereal Diseases," *Canadian Journal of Medicine and Surgery* 21:5 (1908): 301–10; and Power and Murphy, *A System of Syphilis*.

79. "The Routine Treatment of Syphilis," *American Journal of Dermatology and Genito-Urinary Disease* 14 :7 (1910): 355–56; Grover W. Wende, "Dermatology as a Specialty, and Its Relation to Internal Medicine," in *Transactions of the Section on Dermatology of the American Medical Association* (Chicago: American Medical Association Press, 1910), 23.

80. "The Routine Treatment of Syphilis."

81. J. B. Jones, "Moot Points in Syphilis," *Kansas City Medical-Index Lancet* 7:78 (1886): 383; G. M. Phillips, "When to Begin the Specific Treatment of Syphilis," *Hot Springs Medical Journal* 6:5 (1897): 161; "The Routine Treatment of Syphilis"; Fournier, *The Treatment of Syphilis*, 267.

82. H. F. Adams, "Transmission of Syphilis by Parentage or by Inheritance," *Medical Brief* 10:1 (1882): 134–35.

83. He had been dealing with the sore throat for some time. In a letter dated October 1, 1905, he wrote to a friend that "the left side is swollen full, with a big sore back of the tonsil. At times I can hardly swallow. Has been that way for months."

84. "The Thermomineral Cure in the Treatment of Syphilis," *Medicine* 4:7 (1898): 603. See also Irving D. Steinhardt, "The Responsibility of Curing Venereal Diseases," *American Journal of Dermatology and Genito-Urinary Diseases* 14:6 (1910): 282–85; and John H. Stokes, *The Third Great Plague: A Discussion of Syphilis for Everyday People* (Philadelphia: W. B. Saunders, 1918), 145.

85. For evidence of this, see Prince A. Morrow, "Report of the Committee of Seven of the Medical Society of the County of New York on the Prophylaxis of Venereal Disease in New York City," *New York Medical Journal*, December 21, 1910, 1145–50, and December 28, 1910, 1187–92; "Prevalence of Syphilis," *Medical Standard* 28:12 (1901): 670–71; S. Chester Parker, ed., *Yearbook of the National Society for the Study of Education*, vol. 8 (Chicago: University of Chicago Press, 1907), 31; William House, "The Prophylaxis of Syphilis and Its

Sequelae," *Carolina Medical Journal* 53:2 (1905): 571–75; L. Duncan Bulkley, "Analysis of 8,000 Cases of Skin Disease," *Archives of Dermatology* 8 (October 1882): 289–318; and B. Sachs, "Syphilis of the Nervous System," *New York Polyclinic* 2:4 (1893): 75–84. For evidence of the moral fervor that imbued contemporary discussions of the venereal diseases, see J. William White, "The Prevention of Syphilis," *Philadelphia Medical Times*, January 14, 1882, 234–35; and "The Prophylaxis of Venereal Disease," *Occidental Medical Times* 16:7 (1902): 298–99.

86. Keller, "The Hot Springs of Arkansas as a Health Resort," 89.

87. Richard Dewey, "The Mental Condition of John Hart, the Double-Sororicide," *North American Practitioner* 6 (August 1894): 340.

88. William P. Munn, "Treatment of Syphilis," in *Transactions of the Colorado State Medical Society, Thirteenth Annual Convention* (Denver: Colorado State Medical Society, 1900), 325.

89. W. S. Horn, "Treatment of Syphilis at Hot Springs, Arkansas," *United States Navy Medical Bulletin* 4:2 (1910): 155.

90. Lackey, "The Hot Springs of Arkansas," 9.

91. "Hot Springs; the World's Greatest of Health Resorts," *Hot Springs Daily News*, January 17, 1894; *Report of the Secretary of the Interior* (Washington, DC: Government Printing Office, 1885), 880.

92. Loyd Thompson, "The Vale of Healing Waters: An Epic of the Hot Springs of Arkansas," *Medical Pickwick* 6:4 (1920): 135–37.

93. Charles H. Lothrop, *The Remedial Properties of the Hot Springs, Ark.* (St. Louis, MO: Times Printing House, 1881), 82; Randolph Brunson, "Address of Welcome to the Arkansas Medical Society during its Annual Meeting at Hot Springs, May 14, 15, and 16, 1901," *Hot Springs Medical Journal* 10:5 (1901): 163.

94. Thompson, "The Vale of Hot Springs," 135; James T. Jelks, "Treatment of Syphilis at Hot Springs, Arkansas," *Medical News* January 26, 1901, 125.

95. Lackey, "The Hot Springs of Arkansas," 9, emphasis added.

96. W. E. Reynolds, "Hot Springs, Ark.," *Mixer and Server* 22:4 (1913): 41. See also *Transactions of the Grand Lodge of Free and Accepted Masons of the State of Michigan* (Grand Rapids, MI: Grand Lodge, 1912), 102.

97. Orvis Biggs, "The Story of Hot Springs," *Memphis Medical Monthly* 28:12 (1908): 647–48.

98. As the eminent venereal specialist August Ravogli put it, the benefits of a trip to Hot Springs were "in part imaginary"; "like it is for others who go to Lourdes," he surmised, much of this southern city's therapeutic nature derived not from the baths "but rather from the surroundings" ("The Thermomineral Cure in the Treatment of Syphilis," 276).

99. Selden H. Talcott, "Spots on the Spine," *Hahnemannian Monthly* 35 (September 1900): 575.

100. "Influence of the Hot Springs of Arkansas on Syphilis," *Columbus Medical Journal* 8:10 (1890): 458.

101. R. W. Taylor, "The Hot Springs of Arkansas and the Treatment of Syphilis," *Medical Record* April 26, 1890, 464, emphasis added.

102. For information on Francis Schlatter, see A. B. Hyde, "Francis Schlatter, 'the Healer,'" *Chautauquan* 22:4 (1896): 431–35.

103. For examples of these, see George Henry Fox, "The Overtreatment of Syphilis," *Therapeutic Gazette*, 3rd ser., 22:8 (1906): 505–9; Ravogli, *Syphilis in its Medical, Medico-Legal, and Sociological Aspects*, 67; and "A 'Fasting Cure' for Syphilis," *Medico-Pharmaceutical Critic and Guide* 12:2 (1909): 55.

104. George Luys, *A Text-Book on Gonorrhea and Its Complications*, trans. Arthur Foerster (New York: William Wood, 1913), ix–x.

105. E. R. Lewis, "The Hot Springs of Arkansas," *Hot Springs Medical Journal* 2:12 (1893): 276.

106. Talcott, "Spots on the Spine," 575.

107. For more references along these lines, see "Hot Springs," *Medical Mirror*, May 1, 1891, 243–48; and R. W. Taylor, *A Practical Treatise on Genito-Urinary and Venereal Diseases and Syphilis* (New York: Lea Brothers, 1900), 659.

108. For more on this, see Alfred Martin, "The Patron Saint of Syphilis and the Pilgrimage of Syphilitics," *Urologic and Cutaneous Review* 27:2 (1923): 69–82.

109. *The Bibliotheca Sacra*, ed. G. Frederick Wright (Oberlin, OH: Bibliotheca Sacra Company, 1900), 382.

110. Edward F. Wells, "Locomotor Ataxia," *Illinois Medical Journal* 9 (February 1906): 166. For another relevant example, see "Arsenic in the Treatment of Arthritis," *Half-Yearly Compendium of Medical Science* 43:6 (1886): 316–17.

111. James Jelks, "The Hot Springs of Arkansas," in *On the Track and Off the Train*, ed. Lura E. Brown (Little Rock, AR: Press Printing Company, 1892), 176.

112. L. E. Russell, "The Virtues of Hot Springs, Arkansas," *American Medical Journal* 25:3 (1897): 112.

113. "Report of the Superintendent of the Hot Springs Reservation," *Annual Reports of the Department of the Interior for the Fiscal Year Ended June 30, 1903* (Washington, DC: Government Printing Office, 1903), 487.

114. "Hot Springs Reservation, Ark.," *Hearings before Subcommittee of House Committee on Appropriations in Charge of Sundry Civil Appropriation Bill for 1914* (Washington, DC: Government Printing Office, 1914), 782–83.

115. McMechan, "The Hot Springs of Arkansas," 128.

116. Russell, "The Virtues of Hot Springs, Arkansas," 112.

117. Douglas Peter Mackaman, *Leisure Settings: Bourgeois Culture, Medicine, and the Spa in Modern France* (Chicago: University of Chicago Press, 1998), 4.

118. Mackaman, *Leisure Settings*, 113. Another infamous piece of hydrotherapeutic technology from this period was a device popularly known as the "showers of hell," which introduced bathers to a hot, very pressurized form of water. The intense humidity and stench of these waters (which were often sulfuric or alkali in composition) often made it difficult to breathe. See Mackaman, *Leisure Settings*, 110–11.

119. Jelks, "The Hot Springs of Arkansas," 176.

120. Susan Sontag, *AIDS and Its Metaphors* (New York: Farrar, Straus and Giroux, 1989), 101.

121. The origins of this interpretation date back to the work of Susan Sontag, including *Illness as Metaphor* (New York: Farrar, Straus and Giroux, 1978) and *AIDS and Its Metaphors*.

122. For a similar argument along these lines, see Barbara Clow, "Who's Afraid of Susan Sontag? Or, the Myths and Metaphors of Cancer Reconsidered," *Social History of Medicine* 14:2 (2001): 293–312.

123. For an example of this, consider the case of an anonymous English widow suffering from a syphilitic infection contracted via the "intemperate habits" of her late husband. After being admitted to an asylum in 1897, she informed her medical handlers that she was "not doing God's will" and refused medical treatment on the grounds that she "had been ordered to do so by the Almighty as a punishment for her sins." Evidently convinced that her divinely ordained disease could only be cured by religious means, the woman consulted a faith healer and upon leaving the asylum some months later wrote of how she had been "cured by faith[,] . . . saying that the Lord would not allow her to fall." For the details of this case, see Francis O. Simpson, "A Case of Tabes Dorsalis, with Delusional Insanity," *Journal of Nervous and Mental Disease* 24:7 (1897): 409–12.

124. For an example of this, see Antje Kampf, *Mapping out the Venereal Wilderness: Public Health and STD in New Zealand* (London: Transaction, 2007).

125. Keyes, "Influence of the Hot Springs in Arkansas on Syphilis," 64.

126. The finding aid for the Archie A. Cowles papers at the Ohio Historical Society notes that nothing is known of Cowles's life after 1908; the Find a Grave Memorial website (https://www.findagrave.com/memorial/88137380/archie-augustus-cowles) indicates that he died in 1910 and is buried in Charndon, Ohio, but the information does not specific where he died.

127. Special thanks to the Garland County Historical Society for compiling this information.

128. As a navy surgeon familiar with the area put it, Hot Springs' popularity had to do with the fact that "the patient does not have to conceal his disease from everyone, and is not in constant dread that his ailment will be discovered and he disgraced" (Horn, "Treatment of Syphilis at Hot Springs, Arkansas," 155).

129. "I find that a good share of the blind people who come here lost their sight from the kind of catarrh I have," Cowles wrote on August 24, 1907. "Some get their sight back. Some never do."

130. Charles Cutter, *Cutter's Guide to the Hot Springs of Arkansas* (St. Louis, MO: Slawson, 1885), 25. See also G. O. Hebert, "Venereal Prophylaxis," *Journal of Arkansas Medical Society* 6:4 (1909): 105.

131. For a recent reinterpretation of the "white slavery" scare, see Mara L. Keire, *For Business and Pleasure: Red-Light Districts and the Regulation of Vice in the United States, 1890–1933* (Baltimore, MD: Johns Hopkins University Press, 2010).

132. Eugene Carson, "The Advantages in the Treatment of Syphilis at the Hot Springs of Arkansas," *Journal of the American Medical Association* 28:6 (1897): 252.

133. Carson, "The Advantages in the Treatment of Syphilis at the Hot Springs of Arkansas," 252.

134. W. H. Philips, "Hydrotherapy," *Columbus Medical Journal* 2:9 (1884): 393, emphasis added.

Chapter 2 · *"Administering to Minds Diseased"*

1. The story of Michael J. Murphy's visit to Hot Springs comes from an edited collection of his personal correspondence called *The Waiting—A True Love Story: The Last Days of Michael J. Murphy*. The volume was assembled by two of Murphy's descendants, Mary E. Murphy-Hoffman and Lynn Hoffman and can be found at the archives of the National Park Service in Hot Springs, Arkansas. For Murphy's letter of August 5, 1904, see *The Waiting*, 27.

2. Loyd Thompson, "Syphilis and Its Relation to Public Health," *Southern Medical Journal* 9:10 (1916): 882.

3. Allan Brandt, *No Magic Bullet: Venereal Disease and American Society since 1880* (New York: Oxford University, 1987), 5.

4. For examples of this within the literature, see Elizabeth Fee, "Sin vs. Science: Venereal Disease in Baltimore in the Twentieth Century," *Journal of the History of Medicine and Allied Sciences* 43:2 (1988): 158; Brandt, *No Magic Bullet*; Suzanne Poirier, *Chicago's War on Syphilis, 1937–40: The Times, the "Trib," and the Clap Doctor* (Urbana: University of Illinois Press, 1995); Nancy K. Bristow, *Making Men Moral: Social Engineering during the Great War* (New York: New York University Press, 1996); Andrea Tone, *Devices and Desires: A History of Contraceptives in America* (New York: Hill and Wang, 2000); Marilyn Hegarty, *Victory Girls, Khaki-Wackies, and Patriotutes: The Regulation of Female Sexuality during World War Two* (New York: New York University Press, 2008); and John Parascandola, *Sex, Sin, and Science: A History of Syphilis in America* (Westport, CT: Praeger, 2008).

5. For a discussion of this phrase, see James Jones, *Bad Blood: The Tuskegee Syphilis Experiment* (New York: Free Press, 1981).

6. For a similarly complex argument about the relationship between race and medicine in the turn-of-the-century American South, see Christopher Crenner, "Race and Medical Practice in Kansas City's Free Dispensary," *Bulletin of the History of Medicine* 82:4 (2008): 820–46.

7. Oliver C. Wenger, "The Early Days in Hot Springs, Arkansas," Oliver C. Wenger Papers, University of Arkansas for Medical Sciences Archives. As an example of this, consider the career of William H. Barry. Born in Spartansburg, South Carolina, Barry graduated from Memphis Medical College in 1861 and served as a surgeon in the First Arkansas Regiment during the Civil War. In 1875, he moved to Hot Springs, later serving as a president of the state medical society, a member of the state legislature, and chairman of the city board of health. For more on his career, see Fred W. Allsopp, *History of the Arkansas Press for a Hundred Years and More* (Little Rock, AR: Parke-Harpe Publishing Company, 1922), 539.

8. For a complete list of practitioners in Hot Springs during this time, see "Garland County," in *Transactions of the State Medical Society of Arkansas*, vol. 1 (Little Rock, AR: Blochell and Mitchell, 1876), 33.

9. See James T. Jelks, "Treatment of Syphilis at Hot Springs, Arkansas," *Medical News*, January 26, 1901, 124–26.

10. "The Meeting of the American Medical Association," *Occidental Medical Times* 5:6 (1891): 358; "The Latest Organization and Changes in Officers of Sections of the Proposed Ninth International Medical Congress," *Boston Medical and Surgical Journal*, July 9, 1885, 44–45.

11. "One of the fairest dissertations upon the therapeutic value of the Hot Springs," the renowned urologist G. Frank Lydston exclaimed the year after Keller's death, "is an article by Dr. James Keller, whose experience at that resort has certainly been extensive enough to give authority to his opinion" (*The Surgical Diseases of the Genito-Urinary Tract* [Philadelphia: F. A. Davis, 1906], 511).

12. Hal C. Wyman, "A Surgical Pilgrimage to Arkansas," *Physician and Surgeon* 28:5 (1906): 200.

13. "The Negro Physician," *Medical Standard* 21:1 (1898): 2.

14. "The Negro Physician," 3.

15. "Editor's Notes," *American Medico-Surgical Bulletin* 12 (1898): 638.

16. "The Negro Physician," 3.

17. "Arkansas," *Journal of the American Medical Association* 57:14 (1911): 1141. This institution, run by a fraternal order known as the Knights of Pythias, did also admit white patients. See Wyman, "A Surgical Pilgrimage to Arkansas," 200.

18. C. Melnotte Wade, "The Arkansas Hot Springs Baths," *Journal of the National Medical Association* 12:1 (1920): 13–16.

19. C. Melnotte Wade, "Hot Springs—Its People," *Colored American Magazine* 10:1 (1906): 15.

20. For examples of this language, see "Conner's Blood Remedy," *Hot Springs Sentinel-Record*, August 6, 1907, and "Lower Hot Springs Blood Remedy," in Charles Cutter, *Cutter's Guide to Hot Springs* (St. Louis, MO: Slawson, 1900). For more on these medicines, see "Miscellaneous Nostrums," in *Nostrums and Quackery: Articles on the Nostrum Evil and Quackery*, ed. Arthur J. Cramp (Chicago: American Medical Association Press, 1921), 605.

21. According to the makers of one venereal nostrum, mercurial compounds would not only destroy a patient's sense of smell but also "completely derange the whole system." "The damage they will do," an advertisement for Hall's Catarrh Cure (manufactured in Toledo, Ohio) exclaimed, "is ten fold to the good you can possibly derive from them" ("Beware of Ointments for Catarrh That Contain Mercury," *Hot Springs Daily News*, January 17, 1894). Archie Cowles's attraction to Salvar, which he described in a November 10, 1907, letter (Garland County Historical Society, Hot Springs, AR) likely had something to do with the claims of its makers, who publicly proclaimed that it "does not contain Mercury, Potash, Arsenic, Strychnine, nor any Mineral or Opiate in any form or character" ("Salvar Cures," *Hot Springs Sentinel Record*, March 13, 1908).

22. J. H. Marsh, "Are We Doing Our Duty to Prevent the Spread of Venereal Diseases?" in *Transactions of the Medical Society of the State of North Carolina* (Raleigh, NC: Edwards and Broughton, 1906), 597. A 1911 report field by the medical director of the Hot Springs Reservation distressingly concurred, finding a "lucrative field for their operations" there ("Report of the Medical Director of the Hot Springs Reservation, Arkansas," in *Reports of the Department of the Interior, for the Fiscal Year That Ended June 30, 1911* [Washington, DC: Government Printing Office, 1912], 756).

23. *Excluding Advertisements of Cures for Venereal Diseases from the Mails; Hearings before the Committee on the Post Office and Post Roads of the House of Representatives*, 66th Congress (Washington, DC: Government Printing Office, 1919), 24.

24. "Observations at Hot Springs, Arkansas," *Medical and Surgical Reporter*, January 29, 1881, 138.

25. For the complete story of this controversy, see W. David Baird, *Medical Education in Arkansas, 1879–1978* (Memphis, TN: Memphis State University Press, 1979), 16–18.

26. Mrs. Turner Wooton, "Pioneer Doctors of Garland County," *Journal of the Arkansas Medical Society* 46:7 (1949): 143.

27. "Appendix," in *Transactions of the State Medical Society of Arkansas*, 28–29.

28. "Appendix," 22.

29. "Appendix," 24.

30. "Appendix," 28.

31. Wooton, "Pioneer Doctors of Garland County," 143.

32. "Medical News," *Gaillard's Medical Journal* 25:2 (1878): 198–99.

33. For these, see "Physicians, Dentists," *Hot Springs Daily Gazette*, February 24, 1893; "T. J. Reid, M.D.," *Hot Springs Illustrated Monthly* 3:3 (1879): 5.

34. "Professional," *Hot Springs Daily Times*, July 27, 1880.

35. For more on drumming, see chapter 1. Speaking to the ubiquity of this practice, while on his way to Hot Springs, Archie Cowles observed in a July 10, 1907, letter that "if one appears any ways [sic] sick he can hardly reach the Springs without meeting up with a pigeon or so."

36. "Observations at Hot Springs, Arkansas," 137–38. In 1900, one prominent Chicago gynecologist complained that only "about one in ten" of the syphilitic patients he sent to Hot Springs arrived at the office of the "reputable physician" he had directed them to. Once in town, the typical syphilitic was "quite likely to give ear to the wily drummer or the still wilier quack" (Lydston, *The Surgical Diseases of the Genito-Urinary Tract*, 511).

37. *Report of the Medical Director of the Hot Springs Reservation, Arkansas* (Washington, DC: Government Printing Office, 1912), 756–57.

38. "Editor's Notes," *Memphis Medical Monthly* 23:7 (1903): 389.

39. "Editorial Notes," *Kansas City Medical-Index Lancet* 24 (1903): 372; "All We Can, With Your Help," *Hot Springs Medical Journal* 1:3 (1892): 61.

40. "Editor's Notes," 389.

41. "Hot Springs, Arkansas," *Medical Visitor* 20:4 (1904): 141.

42. "Hot Springs, Arkansas," 141.

43. "Hot Springs, Arkansas," 141.

44. Paul T. Vaughan, "Some Observations upon the Ocular Symptoms in Locomotor Ataxia," *Transactions of the State Medical Society of Arkansas* (Little Rock: Arkansas Democrat Co., 1900), 295; James C. Minor, "Urethral Strictures," *Hot Springs Medical Journal* 3:6 (1894): 166.

45. A. L. Elcan, "Syphilis, From a Sanitary and Legal Point of View," *Memphis Medical Monthly* 18:2 (1897): 66; "Proceedings and Discussions at the Seventh Annual Meeting," *Public Health Papers and Reports*, vol. 5 (Boston: Houghton, Mifflin, 1879), 184; Paul T. Vaughan, "Some Remarks Upon Syphilitic Manifestations in the Larynx," *Atlanta Medical and Surgical Journal* 15:4 (1898): 223.

46. Jelks, "Treatment of Syphilis at Hot Springs, Arkansas," 126.

47. According to one local healer, there was "no hope for the syphilitic at present except in mercury and the iodides" (Algernon S. Garnett, "The Dangers of Syphilis and How to Avoid Them," *Hot Springs Medical Journal* 5:3 [1896]: 79–80).

48. M. G. Thompson, "Mercury in the Treatment of Syphilis," *Hot Springs Medical Journal* 1:3 (1892): 51.

49. Loyd Thompson, *Syphilis* (Philadelphia: Lea and Febiger, 1920), 220–21.

50. Edward L. Keyes and Charles H. Chetwood, *Venereal Diseases: Their Complications and Sequelae* (New York: William Wood, 1900), 226.

51. One of the first references to "negro attendants" in Hot Springs comes from a paper published in the late 1870s, which notes that many of these bathhouse employees "have become by long practice very expert as rubbers." See "Hot Springs of Arkansas," *Phrenological Journal* 68:2 (1879): 38. For additional references to black "mercury rubbers," see G. W. Morrison, "The 'Fountains of Perpetual Youth,'" *Four-Track News* 5:5 (1903): 312;

J. M. Thurston, *The Philosophy of Physiomedicalism: Its Theory, Corollary, and Laws of Application in the Cure of Disease* (Richmond, IN: Nicholson Printing, 1900), 361.

52. John C. Paige and Laura Soulliere Harrison, *Out of the Vapors: A Social and Architectural History of Bathhouse Row* (Washington, D.C.: National Park Service, 1988), 136.

53. "Hot Springs Reservation, Ark.," *Hearings before Subcommittee of House Committee on Appropriations in Charge of the Sundry Civil Appropriation Bill for 1914* (Washington, DC: Government Printing Office, 1913), 769–88.

54. "Hot Springs of Arkansas," 37–38.

55. *Nathaniel Price vs. the Standard Life & Accident Insurance Company, Records and Briefs in Cases Decided by the Supreme Court of Minnesota* (April term, 1903), 168.

56. *Nathaniel Price vs. the Standard Life & Accident Insurance Company*, 176.

57. *Nathaniel Price vs. the Standard Life & Accident Insurance Company*, 179.

58. *Nathaniel Price vs. the Standard Life & Accident Insurance Company*, 172.

59. *Nathaniel Price vs. the Standard Life & Accident Insurance Company*, 179.

60. *Nathaniel Price vs. the Standard Life & Accident Insurance Company*, 228.

61. M. R. Richards, "The Hot Baths at Hot Springs," *American Medicine* 14 (1908): 477.

62. *Nathaniel Price vs. the Standard Life & Accident Insurance Company*, 476. For the reference to "strong-armed" attendants, see. Morrison, "The 'Fountains of Perpetual Youth,'" 311–12.

63. "Hot Springs Reservation, Ark.," 764. Typically, bathers paid attendants a fee of $1 per week; the rubbing of mercury incurred an "extra charge" (E. H. Eastman, "Hot Springs, Ark., and Details of the Treatment Given There," *Medical World* 23:9 [1905]: 405).

64. Eugene Carson, "The Comparative Value of the Internal Administration, Inunctions and Injection Method of Administering Mercury in the Treatment of Syphilis," *Journal of the American Medical Association* 53:9 (1909): 676.

65. F. J. Lambkin, *Syphilis: Its Diagnosis and Treatment* (New York: William Wood, 1911), 136; Edward L. Keyes, *The Surgical Diseases of the Genito-Urinary Organs, including Syphilis* (New York: Appleton, 1892), 567.

66. R. C. Corbus, "Four Years' Experience with the Wassermann Reaction in Practice," *Journal of the American Medical Association* 59:14 (1912): 172. See also Arthur Smith Chittenden, "On the Solution of Mercury in the Body," *Philadelphia Medical Journal*, October 28, 1899, 808; George Schuyler Bangert, "Occupational Mercury Poisoning," *New York Medical Journal*, June 22, 1918, 1179–80; and Lavinia Dock, *Text-Book of Materia Medica for Nurses* (New York: G. P. Putnam's Sons, 1890), 40.

67. Paige and Harrison, *Out of the Vapors*, 136.

68. For evidence of this, see "John T. T. Warren," in *The National Cyclopedia of the Colored Race*, ed. Clement Richardson (Montgomery, AL: National Publishing Company, 1919), 382. See also "The Electrical 'Doctor' at Hot Springs," *Western Electrician* 11:1 (1892): 2. For evidence of racism directed against bathhouse attendants, see M. R. Richards, "The Hot Baths at Hot Springs," *American Medicine*, n.s., 3:10 (1908): 475–58; "Hot Springs Reservation, Ark.," 769–88.

69. Charles H. Chetwood, *Genito-Urinary and Venereal Diseases: A Manual for Students and Practitioners* (Philadelphia: Lea Brothers, 1892), 28; Edward L. Keyes, "Cases Bearing Upon Certain Mooted Points in Syphilology," *Medical News*, April 25, 1895, 453.

70. "The Syphilitic and the Hot Bath," *Chicago Clinic* 20:2 (1907): 43.

71. W. S. Horn, "Treatment of Syphilis at Hot Springs, Arkansas," *United States Naval Medical Bulletin* 4:2 (1910): 156.

72. Boasting of the city's "great advantage," resident physicians claimed that "in the treatment of syphilis at Hot Springs . . . the patient can consume a larger amount of mercury and iodides without distressing his system" (Eugene Carson Hay, "Modern Methods of Treating Syphilis," in *Transactions of the Mississippi Valley Medical Association* [Kansas City, MO: Burd and Fletcher, 1903], 278–79).

73. Jelks, "Treatment of Syphilis at Hot Springs, Arkansas," 126.

74. Thompson, "Mercury in the Treatment of Syphilis," 52.

75. T. M. Baird, "The Hygienic Treatment of Syphilis," *Hot Springs Medical Journal* 4:1 (1895): 12.

76. Jelks, "Treatment of Syphilis at Hot Springs, Arkansas," 125.

77. Jelks, "Treatment of Syphilis at Hot Springs, Arkansas," 125.

78. Loyd Thompson, "The Intensive Treatment of Syphilis," *Journal of the American Medical Association* 67:10 (1916): 735.

79. Garnett, "The Dangers of Syphilis and How to Avoid Them," 80.

80. C. Travis Drennen, "Hygiene for the Syphilitic," *Memphis Medical Monthly* 18:2 (1897): 57.

81. M. G. Thompson, "Sexual Disorders and One of the Causes of Unhappy Marriages," *Memphis Medical Monthly* 28:3 (1908): 175; Thompson, "The Intensive Treatment of Syphilis," 735.

82. M. G. Thompson, "Gonorrhea, Its Cause and the Treatment of Some of Its Sequels," *Hot Springs Medical Journal* 1:1 (1892): 9–10; M. G. Thompson, "Impotence in the Male," *Memphis Medical Monthly* 6:2 (1897): 71.

83. Baird, "The Hygienic Treatment of Syphilis," 13.

84. Thompson, "Impotence in the Male," 71.

85. James T. Jelks, "The Antiquity of Syphilis, and Moses as a Health Officer," *Journal of the American Medical Association* 21:4 (1893): 108.

86. Jelks, "The Antiquity of Syphilis, and Moses as a Health Officer," 109.

87. Jelks, "The Antiquity of Syphilis, and Moses as a Health Officer," 109.

88. Jelks, "Treatment of Syphilis at Hot Springs, Arkansas," 125; Charles Dake, "The Treatment of Syphilis," *Southern Journal of Homeopathy* 10:9 (1892): 906.

89. Jelks, "Treatment of Syphilis at Hot Springs, Arkansas," 125.

90. James C. Minor, "Rest as a Therapeutic Agent," *Hot Springs Medical Journal* 2:4 (1893): 75.

91. Robert W. Taylor, *A Practical Treatise on Genito-Urinary and Venereal Diseases and Syphilis* (New York: Lea Brothers, 1900), 639.

92. Bukk G. Carleton, *A Treatise on Urological and Venereal Diseases and Venereal Diseases* (Philadelphia: Boericke and Tafel, 1905), 741.

93. Henry W. Stelwagon, *Treatise on the Diseases of the Skin* (Philadelphia: W. B. Saunders, 1910), 814.

94. James W. White and Edward H. Martin, *White and Martin's Genito-Urinary Surgery and Venereal Diseases* (Philadelphia: J. B. Lippincott, 1918), 883. See also Edward L. Keyes, "Influence of the Hot Springs in Arkansas on Syphilis," *Journal of Cutaneous and Genito-Urinary Diseases* 8:2 (1890): 63–68.

95. R. W. Taylor, "The Hot Springs of Arkansas and the Treatment of Syphilis," *Medical Record* April 26, 1890, 463. See also L. D. Bulkley, "What Real Value Have the Natural Mineral Waters in the Treatment of Diseases of the Skin," *Boston Medical and Surgical Journal*, October 10, 1889, 368.

96. "The Syphilitic and the Hot Bath," 43.

97. "Simple Thermal Waters in the Treatment of Syphilis," *Chicago Clinic* 21:7 (1908): 203.

98. Everett Myers, "Syphilis and Problems in Its Prevention," *Journal of the Arkansas Medical Society* 8:3 (1911): 80. For more on local doctors' attitudes toward male sexuality, see G. O. Hebert, "Venereal Prophylaxis," *Journal of the Arkansas Medical Society* 6:4 (1909): 114–18; and Thomas Douglass, "Erotomania," *Journal of the Arkansas Medical Society* 13:4 (1916): 67–75.

99. Thompson, "Sexual Disorders and One of the Causes of Unhappy Marriages," 175.

100. Steven M. Stowe, *Doctoring the South: Southern Physicians and Everyday Medicine in the Mid-Nineteenth Century* (Chapel Hill: University of North Carolina Press, 2004), 93.

101. Stowe, *Doctoring the South*, 263.

102. Samuel Pye, "The Hot Springs of Arkansas," *Christian Advocate*, March 9, 1899, 384.

103. "To Reform Hot Springs," *Medical News*, July 8, 1905, 83.

104. "To Reform Hot Springs," 83; Pye, "The Hot Springs of Arkansas," 384.

105. "Arkansas Department," *Meyer Brothers Druggist* 19:6 (1898), 401.

106. Pye, "The Hot Springs of Arkansas," 384.

107. For more on this, see Philip K. Wilson, "Bad Habits and Bad Genes: Early 20th-Century Eugenic Attempts to Eliminate Syphilis and Associated 'Defects' from the United States," *Canadian Bulletin of the History of Medicine* 20:1 (2003): 20.

108. For more on this phrase, see Jones, *Bad Blood*. Most southern physicians agreed that "the prevalence of syphilis in the negro is so marked that it is customary to regard each individual as syphilitic until proved otherwise" (William C. Sandy, "Syphilis in Relation to Mental Disease," *International Record of Medicine and General Practice Clinics*, April 20, 1918, 734).

109. T. LeRoy Jefferson, "Syphilis and Tuberculosis in the Negro," *Medical World* 28:7 (1910): 292; Thomas W Murrell, "Syphilis and the American Negro: A Medico-Sociological Study," in *Transactions of the Fortieth Annual Session of the Medical Society of Virginia* 40 (Richmond, VA: Everett Waddey,1909), 168. As one Alabama doctor had it, slavery afforded African Americans "the best hygienic surroundings the world has ever seen" (Seale Harris, "The Future of the Negro from the Standpoint of the Southern Physician," *Alabama Medical Journal* 14:2 [1902]: 63).

110. Jefferson, "Syphilis and Tuberculosis in the Negro," 292; Harris, "The Future of the Negro from the Standpoint of the Southern Physician," 63.

111. Louis Wender, "The Role of Syphilis in the Insane Negro," *New York Medical Journal*, December 30, 1916, 1287; "Discussion on Syphilis," *Journal of the American Medical Association* 63:7 (1914): 565; Charles R. Grandy, "Heart Disease in the Negro, Based on a Study of One-Hundred Cases," in *Transactions of the Forty-Sixth Annual Session of the Medical Society of Virginia* (Richmond, VA: Richmond Press, 1916), 60. See also, "Discussion on Syphilis," 565. Southern medical men often traced the increasing incidence of general paresis of the insane—a tertiary complication of syphilis—to the effects of civilization. For

more on this, see Charles W. Burr, "Civilization and Insanity," *Journal of Sociologic Medicine* 18:5 (1917): 339; Ernest L. Zimmerman, "A Comparative Study of Syphilis in Whites and in Negroes," *Archives of Dermatology and Syphilology* 4:1 (1921): 86; and Leo Kanner, "The Racial Prospect of General Paralysis," *American Journal of Syphilis* 11:1 (1927): 25.

112. For an example of this racialized discourse, see Noel M. Moore, "Hereditary Syphilis in the Negro Race," *Southern Medical Journal* 8:11 (1915): 946–48.

113. When writing about prostitutes, doctors also drew attention to the relative rarity of tabes and paresis among this group of syphilitics, contending that "a large proportion" never experienced that late stage of the disease that primarily affected the brain. Those who did were said to be imbeciles and mental defectives. For more on this, see A. Read Wilson, "Some Rarer Manifestations of Parasyphilis of the Nervous System," *Brain: A Journal of Neurology* 35:2 (1913): 153–89; and F. W. Mott, "On the Causes of Insanity," *Lancet*, July 11, 1914, 75–82.

114. "Syphilis as a Cause of Insanity," *Journal of Mental Sciences* 48:200 (1902): 808; "Exercise and Deterioration in Tabes," *Medical News*, November 7, 1903, 895.

115. E. M. Hummel, "The Rarity of Tabetic and Paretic Conditions in the Negro," *Journal of the American Medical Association* 106:22 (1911): 1646.

116. "Exercise and Deterioration in Tabes," 895.

117. "Exercise and Deterioration in Tabes," 895.

118. George H. Rohe, "Lectures on the Cutaneous Manifestations of Syphilis," *Medical Age* 6:8 (1888): 176.

119. Howard Fox, "A Case of Annular Papular Syphilis in a Negress," *Journal of the American Medical Association* 60:19 (1913): 1420.

120. Frank A. Jones, "Cardiac Lesions as Observed in the Negro, with Special Reference to Pericarditis," *Journal of the American Medical Association* 37:2 (1901): 1582.

121. Hummel, "The Rarity of Tabetic and Paretic Conditions in the Negro," 1646.

122. Jefferson, "Syphilis and Tuberculosis in the Negro," 293.

123. Murrell, "Syphilis and the American Negro," 169–70.

124. Murrell, "Syphilis and the American Negro," 169–70.

125. Murrell, "Syphilis and the American Negro," 169; "Syphilis in the American Negro," *Ohio's Health* 4:8 (1915): 1317.

126. Hummel, "The Rarity of Tabetic and Paretic Conditions in the Negro," 1646.

127. L. R. Ellis, "Address of the Chairman of the Section on Dermatology and Syphilology," *Journal of the Arkansas Medical Society* 6:2 (1909): 44.

128. Thompson, *Syphilis*, 52; Loyd Thompson and Lyle B. Kingerly, "Syphilis in the Negro," *American Journal of Syphilis, Gonorrhea, and the Venereal Diseases* 3:3 (1919): 396.

129. C. Travis Drennen, "Syphilis as an Aetiological Factor in the Production of Locomotor Ataxis," *Hot Springs Medical Journal* 5:11 (1896): 369.

130. A. W. Hunton, "The American Carlsbad," *Voice of the Negro* 3:5 (1906): 331. For more evidence of racial discrimination at the resort, see "Hot Springs, Arkansas, Wants Help from Uncle Sam," *Colored American Magazine* 12:6 (1907): 409–10.

131. "Negroes Can Bathe at French Lick Springs," *Michigan State News*, Tuskegee Institute news clippings file.

132. For more on Fitzhugh's life, see *Slave Narratives: A Folk History of Slavery in the United States from Interviews with Former Slaves*, vol. 2, *Arkansas*, pt. 2, Cannon-Evans (Washington, DC: Government Printing Office, 1941), 305–11.

133. *A Folk History of Slavery in the United States from Interviews with Former Slaves*, 307.

134. John A. Kenney, *The Negro in Medicine* (Tuskegee, AL: Tuskegee Institute Press, 1912), 91. See also "Medical Schools," *Journal of the National Medical Association* 15:1 (1923): 55.

135. Harold H. Phipps, "The Therapeutics of Hot Springs and Other Mineral Waters of Hot Springs, Arkansas, in the Treatment of Syphilis, Rheumatism, and Other Diseases," *Journal of the National Medical Association* 1:1 (1909): 183.

136. Phipps, "The Therapeutics of Hot Springs and Other Mineral Waters of Hot Springs, Arkansas, in the Treatment of Syphilis, Rheumatism, and Other Diseases," 183. For his part, none of Wade's publications mention syphilis at all. See, for example, C. M. Wade, "The Arkansas Hot Springs Baths," *Journal of the National Medical Association* 12:1 (1920): 13–16.

137. In a presentation given at the 1911 meeting of the National Medical Association, an Alabama doctor discussed a patient with tertiary syphilis who, after years of unsuccessful treatment in Montgomery, was sent to Hot Springs—where he was advised to take "mercury baths in connection with the other Hot Springs treatment." For this case, see U. G. Mason, "Observation: Use and Abuse of Salvarsan," *Journal of the National Medical Association* 3:4 (1911): 340–44.

138. Indeed, within the medical literature authored by white resort doctors, there is but one article mentioning black VD patients in Hot Springs. See Drennen, "Syphilis as an Aeteological Factor in the Production of Locomotor Ataxia," 370.

139. For another account of this, see James Byrd, "African Americans and the Bathhouses of Hot Springs, Arkansas," *Garland County Historical Society Record* 59 (2018): 1–16.

140. "Why Does the Southern Negro Escape the Ravages of Syphilis?" *Southern Practitioner* 27:6 (1905): 349.

141. "Why Does the Southern Negro Escape the Ravages of Syphilis?" 350.

142. Stowe, *Doctoring the South*, 209.

143. Thompson, "Sexual Disorders and One of the Causes of Unhappy Marriages," 175.

144. For more on this, see Paul A. Lombardo and Gregory Dorr, "Eugenics, Medical Education, and the Public Health Service: Another Perspective on the Tuskegee Syphilis Experiment," *Bulletin of the History of Medicine* 80:2 (2006): 291–316.

145. For a recent discussion of these developments, see Paul Lombardo, "A Child's Right to Be Born: Venereal Disease and the Eugenic Marriage Laws, 1913–1935," *Perspectives in Biology and Medicine* 60:2 (2017): 211–32.

146. Wilson, "Bad Habits and Bad Genes."

147. Drennen, "Syphilis as an Aeteological Factor in the Production of Locomotor Ataxia," 367.

148. Frederick L. Hoffman, *A Plan for a More Effective Federal and State Health Administration* (Newark, NJ: Prudential Press, 1919), 80.

149. "America's Mid-Continental Playground—Hot Springs, Ark.," *South-West* 5:1 (1906): 19. The concept of neurasthenia was popularized by American neurologist George Beard, whose book *American Nervousness: Its Causes and Consequences* (New York: G. P. Putnam's Sons) declared the disorder the result of middle- and upper-class workers' inability to cope with "the great mental activity made necessary and possible in a new and productive country" (7–8).

150. Brad Campbell, "The Making of 'American': Race and Nation in Neurasthenic Discourse," *History of Psychiatry* 18:2 (2007): 172.

151. Campbell, "The Making of 'American,'" 161.

152. Campbell, "The Making of 'American,'" 174.

153. Charles M. Nice, "Neurasthenia," *Southern Medical Journal* 1:2 (1908): 104–12.

154. Ludwig Bremer, "Current Fallacies about Nervous Prostration," *St. Louis Clinique* 7:4 (1894): 148.

155. Titus M. Coan, "The Curative Uses of Water," *Harper's Magazine* 75:449 (1887): 776. For other endorsements of Hot Springs' therapeutic value in cases of neurasthenia, see I. N. Love, "Neurasthenia," *Journal of the American Medical Association* 22:15 (1894): 544.

156. E. R Lewis, "The Hot Springs of Arkansaw," *Kansas City Medical Index-Lancet* 10:7 (1889): 249); *Report of the Surgeon General* (Washington, DC: Government Printing Office, 1891), 9.

157. E. G. Jones, "The Man Who Sojourneth at Hot Springs," *Western Medical Reporter* 14:6 (1892): 144.

158. "Hot Springs," *Medical Mirror*, May 1, 1891, 246.

159. "Editorial," *Hot Springs Medical Journal* 3:2 (1894): 81.

160. Jelks, "Treatment of Syphilis at Hot Springs, Arkansas," 125.

161. Minor, "Rest as a Therapeutic Agent," 76–77.

162. W. H. Barry, "Healthful Exercise," *Hot Springs Medical Journal* 6:10 (1897): 301.

163. M. G. Thompson, "Some Observations Concerning Rheumatism," *Journal of the Arkansas Medical Society* 5:11 (1908): 278–80.

164. Thompson, "Gonorrhea, Its Cause and the Treatment of Some of Its Sequels," 9.

165. Thompson, "Gonorrhea, Its Cause and the Treatment of Some of Its Sequels," 9.

166. Thompson, "Gonorrhea, Its Cause and the Treatment of Some of Its Sequels," 9–10.

167. Minor, "Rest as a Therapeutic Agent," 76.

168. Thompson, "Gonorrhea, Its Cause and the Treatment of Some of Its Sequels," 9–10.

169. Joseph H. Cloidt, record group 112, AR-6, box 8, Records of Army and Navy General Hospital, Hot Springs, AR, National Archives, Fort Worth, TX.

170. James H. Chesnutt, "Brain Syphilis," *Journal of the Arkansas Medical Society* 7:12 (1911): 293.

171. Chesnutt, "Brain Syphilis," 293.

172. Chesnutt, "Brain Syphilis," 294.

173. Chesnutt, "Brain Syphilis," 294.

174. Gonorrhea was another malady subjected to racial bifurcations. Prior to the discovery of *Neisseria gonorrhoeae* in 1872, doctors believed that gonorrhea was a disease of immigrants and the working poor. Young girls of low socioeconomic status diagnosed with gonorrhea were often said be victims of child rape—that is, of sexual assault at the hands of "ignorant Italians, Chinese, and Negroes" who adhered to the superstitious belief that (as one physician put it) "if a man afflicted with an obstinate VD have intercourse with a virgin, the latter will develop the disease and he will be cured." In the 1890s, improved diagnostic methods led to the recognition that many daughters of the well-to-do also suffered from gonorrhea. Yet instead of concluding that these infections were also the result of rape, doctors insisted that in the case of "respectable" white families, other, nonsexual modes of transmission (like contaminated toilet seats) were to blame. In emphasizing the "innocent" nature of these infections, the medical profession found a way to reduce the social stigma of VD among middle- and upper-class whites and of preserving

their moral integrity. For more on this, see Lynn Sacco, "Sanitized for Your Protection:" Medical Discourse and the Denial of Incest in the United States, 1890–1940," *Journal of Women's History* 14:3 (2002): 84, 87.

175. "The Non-Institutional Treatment of Syphilis," *Journal of Physical Therapy* 1:12 (1905): 564.

176. "The Non-Institutional Treatment of Syphilis," 564.

177. "The Non-Institutional Treatment of Syphilis," 565.

178. "The Non-Institutional Treatment of Syphilis," 566.

179. For additional evidence of Hot Springs' influence on individual practitioners, see J. M. French, "Syphilitic Epilepsy," *Cincinnati Lancet and Clinic*, June 17, 1882, 556–59; and J. T. Warnock, "I Owe My Life to Orificial Surgery," *Journal of Orificial Surgery* 1:4 (1893): 255–60.

180. Whereas some doctors believed that the superiority of Hot Springs lay in doctors' elevation of drugless remedies, others drew the opposite conclusion and pointed out how local healers showed that the shift away from "heroic treatment" with mercury had been a step backward in venereology. For evidence of this view, see Taylor, "The Hot Springs of Arkansas and the Treatment of Syphilis."

181. As a result of these connections, some doctors established referral networks with Hot Springs doctors. For an example of this, see Thomas Kennard, "Round-Celled Sarcoma or Encephaloid Sarcoma—involving the Tibia and the Knee-Joint," *Proceedings of the St. Louis Medical Society of Missouri*, vol. 2 (St. Louis, MO: George O. Rumbold, 1879), 82–86.

182. L. G. LeBeuf, "Syphilis with Notes on Symptomatology, Hygiene and Treatment by the Inunction Method," *New Orleans Medical and Surgical Journal* 60:3 (1907): 219.

Chapter 3 · Diagnosing Syphilis at Army and Navy Hospital

1. For Jones's complete clinical case file, see record group 112.5.1, box 28, Records of Army and Navy General Hospital, Hot Springs, AR, National Archives, Fort Worth, TX. Hereafter cited by box number.

2. Josiah J. Moore, "The Wassermann Test in the Medical Dispensary," *Journal of the American Medical Association* 65:23 (1915): 1983; *United States Naval Medical Bulletin* 5:1 (1911): 443; "The Wassermann Reaction and Its Value to the Physician," *Indianapolis Medical Journal* 13:11 (1910): 536.

3. Ilana Löwy, "The History of the Wassermann Reaction," in *AIDS and Contemporary History*, ed. Virginia Berridge and Philip Strong (New York: Cambridge University Press, 1993), 86. Concurring with this view, Paula Mazumdar has argued that "a positive reaction was as much a sign of syphilis as a skin lesion" ("'In the Silence of the Laboratory': The League of Nations Standardized Syphilis Tests," *Social History of Medicine* 16:3 [2003]: 441).

4. Simon Szreter, "The Prevalence of Syphilis in England and Wales on the Eve of the Great War," *Social History of Medicine* 27:3 (2014): 516; Han Neefs, "The Introduction of Diagnostic and Treatment Innovations for Syphilis in Post-War VD Policy: The Belgian Experience," *Dynamis* 24 (2004): 99.

5. Anne R. Hanley, *Medicine, Knowledge, and Venereal Diseases in England, 1886–1916* (New York: Palgrave MacMillan, 2017), 130.

6. Amy Fairchild, *Science at the Borders: Immigrant Medical Inspection and the Shaping of the Modern Industrial Labor Force* (Baltimore, MD: Johns Hopkins University Press, 2003), 176.

7. Gayle Davis, *"The Cruel Madness of Love":* Sex, Syphilis, and Psychiatry in Scotland, *1880–1930* (New York: Rodopi, 2008), 231.

8. For scholarship generally in favor of this idea, see John Duffy, *A History of Public Health in New York City,* vol. 2 (New York: Russell Sage Foundation, 1974); Morris J. Vogel and Charles Rosenberg, eds., *The Therapeutic Revolution: Essays in the Social History of American Medicine* (Philadelphia: University of Pennsylvania Press, 1979); John Harley Warner, *The Therapeutic Perspective: Medical Practice, Knowledge, and Identity in America, 1820–1885* (Cambridge, MA: Harvard University Press, 1986); and Andrew Cunningham and Perry Williams, eds., *The Laboratory Revolution in Medicine* (New York: Cambridge University Press, 1992). For more on the various "germ theories" circulating through late-nineteenth century medical culture, see Michael Worboys, *Spreading Germs: Disease Theories and Medical Practice in Britain, 1865–1900* (Cambridge: Cambridge University Press, 2000).

9. Henk van den Belt, "The Collective Construction of a Scientific Fact: A Re-Examination of the Early Period of the Wassermann Reaction, 1906–1912," *Social Epistemology* 25:4 (2011): 324.

10. The first work to seriously question the laboratory revolution idea was L. S. Jacyna, "The Laboratory and the Clinic: The Impact of Pathology on Surgical Diseases in the Glasgow Western Infirmary, 1875–1910," *Bulletin of the History of Medicine* 62:3 (1988): 384–406. For more recent revisions of the laboratory revolution thesis, see Charles Hayter, "The Clinic as Laboratory: The Case of Radiation Therapy, 1896–1920," *Bulletin of the History of Medicine* 72:4 (1998): 663–88; Christiane Sinding, "Making the Unit of Insulin: Standards, Clinical Work, and Industry, 1920–25," *Bulletin of the History of Medicine* 76:2 (2002): 231–70; and Davis, *"The Cruel Madness of Love,"* esp. chapter 4. Some of the most up-to-date scholarship on the nature of the relationship between the lab and the clinic in turn-of-the-century medicine has recently been published in *Social History of Medicine* 24:3 (2011); see in particular, Steve Sturdy, "Looking for Trouble: Medical Science and Clinical Practice in the Historiography of Modern Medicine," 739–57; Morten Hammerborg, "The Laboratory and the Clinic Revisited," 758–75; Rosemary Wall, "Using Bacteriology in Elite Hospital Practice: London and Cambridge, 1880–1920," 776–96; and Mirjam Stuij, "Explaining Trends in Body Weight: Offer's Rational and Myopic Choice vs. Elias' Theory of Civilizing Processes," 796–812. See also Elliott Bowen, "Limits of the Lab: Diagnosing 'Latent Gonorrhea,' 1872–1910," *Bulletin of the History of Medicine* 87:1 (2013): 63–85.

11. For more on this, see Charles Rosenberg, *The Care of Strangers: The Rise of America's Hospital System* (New York: Basic Books, 1987).

12. For more on these developments, see Theda Skocpol, *Protecting Soldiers and Mothers: The Origins of Social Policy in the United States* (Cambridge, MA: Harvard University Press, 1992); Ronald Barr, *The Progressive Army: U.S. Army Command and Administration, 1870–1914* (New York: St. Martin's Press, 1998); Roger Possner, *The Rise of Militarism in the Progressive Era, 1900–1914* (Jefferson, NC: McFarland, 2009); and Beth Linker, *War's Waste: Rehabilitation in World War One America* (Chicago: University of Chicago Press, 2011).

13. For more on the growth of the military's hospital system, see Mary C. Gillet, *The Army Medical Department, 1865–1917* (Washington, DC: Center of Military History, US Army, 1995); and Bobby A. Wintermute, *Public Health and the U.S. Military: A History of the Army Medical Department, 1818–1917* (New York: Routledge, 2011).

14. For an informative, up-to-date study on the creation of Walter Reed Hospital, see Jessica L. Adler, "The Founding of Walter Reed Hospital and the Beginnings of Modern Institutional Army Medical Care in the United States," *Journal of the History of Medicine and Allied Sciences* 69:4 (2014): 521–53.

15. For more on this, see Carol R. Byerly. *"Good Tuberculosis Men": The Army Medical Department's Struggle with Tuberculosis* (Fort Sam Houston, TX: Office of the Surgeon General Borden Institute, 2013).

16. See James E. Pilcher, "The Prevention of the Extension of Venereal Disease among Soldiers," *Columbus Medical Journal* 18:5 (1899): 274–76; Valery Havard, "Venereal Diseases in the Army and Their Prophylaxis," *New York State Journal of Medicine* 6:5 (1907): 207–10; and Frank R. Keefer, *A Textbook of Military Hygiene and Sanitation* (Philadelphia: W. B. Saunders, 1914).

17. For evidence of the controversy surrounding this, see "A National Disgrace," *Woman's Column*, November 17, 1900, 1–3.

18. See Charles D. Camp, "Non-Operative Treatment of Bubo," *Medical Brief* 29:1 (1900): 40. For a discussion of the military's attempts at chemical prophylaxis, see Andrea Tone, *Devices and Desires* (New York: Hill and Wang, 2000), esp. chapter 5.

19. "Hospital," *New International Encyclopedia*, vol. 11 (New York: Dodd, Mead, 1915), 503. See also the section on the Army and Navy General Hospital Arkansas," in "Extracts from the Report of the Surgeon-General, United States Army, 1887," *Chicago Medical Journal and Examiner* 56:1 (1888): 35; and "Medical Notes," *Boston Medical and Surgical Journal*, June 15, 1882: 571 (section on Washington).

20. *General Orders and Circulars, Adjutant General's Office* (Washington, DC: Government Printing Office, 1887), 174.

21. *Report of the Surgeon-General of the Army to the Secretary of War for the Fiscal Year Ending 1886* (Washington, DC: Government Printing Office, 1888), 11–12.

22. "The United States Government Hospitals at the Hot Springs," *Medical Record*, March 29, 1890, 357.

23. *Manual of the Medical Department, United States Navy* (Washington, DC: Government Printing Office, 1906), 40, emphasis added.

24. *Manual for the Medical Department, United States Army* (Washington, DC: Government Printing Office, 1900), 44.

25. William P. Philips, box 42. As another example, consider the case of William Nichols, a forty-two-year-old private who in the summer of 1909 found himself bedridden at Vancouver Barracks in Washington State (box 40). On September 8, 1909, a surgeon at this western base camp mailed a letter to the adjutant general (Department of the Columbia) detailing the nature of his patient's disability, which he officially diagnosed as chronic rheumatism. That being the case, the man's attendant had initially considered sending Nichols to the Army and Navy General Hospital, but as the source of this soldier's ailments were "in question," he soon reconsidered the prudence of such a move, noting that "rheumatism of specific nature is not accepted at the Hot Springs." According to the medical officer in charge, although he "disclaimed" it, Nichols "presented some of the manifestations of antecedent syphilis." Therefore, and "in justice to the soldiers and myself," his surgeon ultimately requested a transfer to the General Hospital at the San Francisco Presidio, which had no such antivenereal ban.

26. For an example of this, consider the case of George M. Beatty ("George M. Beatty," *Decisions of the Department of the Interior in Appealed Pension and Bounty-Land Claims*, vol. 13 [Washington, DC: Government Printing Office, 1903], 192–201). An Illinois veteran of the Civil War, Beatty came to the attention of federal authorities in 1903, when he applied to the Commissioner of Pensions for an increase in the monthly stipend allotted to him on account of "rheumatism and resulting disease of left knee and shoulder" (192). Already the recipient of a $30 per month pension, Beatty' was requesting additional compensation because he now required the "regular personal aid and attention of another person" for the care of his continually deteriorating condition. Reviewing Beatty's case, federal officials initially seemed poised to deny his request, especially after learning that he now suffered from locomotor ataxia and general paresis—both common consequences of syphilis. Even though clinical examinations revealed "no objective or subjective history of syphilis," bureau agents suspected a specific origin for Beatty's ailments, noting in particular that prior to being discharged from the army he had been "treated at Hot Springs[,] . . . a place, as is well known, that is eminently well-fitted for the treatment of the disease in question, and that is resorted to by large numbers of persons suffering from such disease" (199). However, when faced with Beatty's stringent denials, as well as the fact that "persons suffering from rheumatism also go there for treatment," the commissioner ultimately relented, approving his increased monthly pension even in the face of his own unresolved doubts and misgivings.

27. W. F. Arnold, "Statistical Methods in Therapeutics," *Military Surgeon* 21:3 (1907): 231.

28. See Augustus Leecing, box 32; Fred M. Jones, box 28; and Charles Lyons, box 33.

29. Anderson Phifer, box 43.

30. The Army and Navy Hospital's case files are organized alphabetically by patient's last name, so each box contains records from different years. It should also be noted here that the figures in the rightmost column do *not* include cases in which doctors rendered ambivalent diagnoses like "Syph?" Given this, the number of patients given antivenereal medicines is higher than the number of patients diagnosed with VD.

31. For other cases like this, see William Ragland, John R. Rauhoff, and Charles D. Reynolds, box 44.

32. James N. Hyde, *A Manual of Syphilis and the Venereal Diseases* (Philadelphia: W. B. Saunders, 1908): 362; Leon L. Solomon, "Group Medicine Diagnosis," *Journal of the Indiana State Medical Association* 15:3 (1922): 87.

33. E. F. Snydacker, "Involvement of the Eye in Syphilis," *Illinois Medical Journal* 9 (April 1906): 420; Landon Carter Gray, "The Diagnosis of One Form of Intra-Cranial Syphilis," *American Journal of Medical Sciences* 103 (January 1892): 31.

34. George Stopford-Taylor and Robert W. Mackenna, *The Salvarsan Treatment of Syphilis in Private Practice* (London: William Heinemann, 1914), 17–18.

35. Solomon, "Group Medicine Diagnosis," 87.

36. For additional cases like Lepphardt's, see Charles E. Johnston, box 28, Peter Holden, box 25, Bruin D. Mead, box 37, and Henry Harrig, box 23.

37. For evidence of this, see Roy Oliver, box 41, Dell Hart, box 23, David Hamilton, box 23, and William Mitchell, box 38.

38. Nathaniel B. Potter and James C. Wilson, *Internal Medicine*, vol. 2 (Philadelphia: J. B. Lippincott, 1919), 226. See also R. E. McVey, "Syphilis," *Kansas Medical Journal*, April 17, 1897, 212.

39. Well into the 1920s, doctors continued to acknowledge the Wassermann's weakness with respect to syphilis's late-stage complications; "in tertiary syphilis it is very frequently only mildly positive," one specialist said of the serological test, adding that it was "sometimes negative" (E. E. Butler, "The Diagnosis of Tertiary Syphilis," *Kentucky Medical Journal* 20:8 [1922]: 517, 519).

40. Byrom Bramwell, "The Etiological Relationship of Syphilis to Tabes and General Paresis of the Insane," *Clinical Studies* 4:2 (1906): 97–116.

41. William A. Pusey, *The Principles and Practice of Dermatology* (New York: Appleton, 1907): 573.

42. The shockingly open and revealing testimony provided by Morris Haddox led Army and Navy surgeons toward a relatively straightforward and simple venereal diagnosis. Admitted to the hospital in March 1900, Haddox immediately disclosed that during the previous winter he had noticed a "chancre" on his penis; a body rash, sore throat, and an ulcer on the tongue soon followed. After hearing of this and taking into account their patient's statement that he had "been taking mercury pills by mouth and also potassium iodide since February," Haddox's medical attendants diagnosed him with secondary syphilis and immediately continued the antisyphilitic regimen he had embarked on. By late January of 1901, he had been "cured" and returned to duty (box 24).

43. For examples of this, see Bruin D. Mead, box 37; Peter Holden, box 25; and Dell Hart, box 23.

44. Rhodes was not the only patient who may have resorted to subterfuge in order to gain admittance to the hospital. For example, when Charles McCracken entered Army and Navy on October 17, 1901, with a "scar on [the] glans penis," he insisted that this was the result of an accident in which he "fell on a ladder and mashed [the] end of [his] penis"—the presence of "numerous gonococci" in his urine notwithstanding. At first, the ruse seemed to work, but after a few days, McCracken was discharged "for gonorrheal rheumatism and chronic gonorrhea . . . not in the line of duty" (box 35).

45. For a similar case, see Robert Nicholson, box 38.

46. One early twentieth-century venereal specialist, referring to syphilis of the tongue, proclaimed that "diagnosis from cancer and tuberculosis may be difficult, and may require a therapeutic test with anti-syphilitic treatment before a positive conclusion can be reached" (Edgar G. Ballenger and James E. Paullin, *Genito-Urinary Diseases and Syphilis* [Atlanta: E. W. Allen, 1913], 408).

47. J. M. Koch, "The Diagnosis of Acquired Secondary Syphilis Where the History and Initial Lesion are Absent," *Medical Bulletin* 17:11 (1895): 413.

48. KI is the chemical formula for potassium iodide, according to the periodic table of elements.

49. Another patient subjected to the procedure was James Oden. Suffering from stiffness and pains in his joints, Oden was transferred to Hot Springs from Fort Howard, Maryland, on February 19, 1904, where he initially received a diagnosis of myalgia, for which doctors prescribed a standard course of baths. One month later, however, a mercurial unguent was applied to his skin. For the next week, doctors administered this anti-syphilitic remedy on a daily basis. Then, without any explanation, they returned to the earlier course of treatment for myalgia. What prompted this short-lived foray into venereal medication, it seems, was Oden's physical symptoms, as he exhibited sores "over the chest and arms strongly suggestive of syphilis." Such signs prompted resident surgeons

to experiment with antivenereal drugs, though their syphilitic suspicions apparently proved unfounded in the long run (box 38).

50. For examples of doctors' use of the "therapeutic test," see Roy Oliver, box 41; August Hartell, box 23; and Robert Hudson, box 27.

51. For more cases like these, see Frederick C. Kidd, box 30; Thomas E. Mayo, box 35; and Jay Lane, box 31.

52. Cyrus Jackson, box 30; Jay Lane, box 31; William B. Fuhrer, box 19.

53. This was something that local practitioners freely admitted. "The differential signs between eczema and syphilis of the palms and soles, so far as the objective appearances go, are very obscure," declared the Hot Springs practitioner John A. Fordyce in a 1906 article, adding that "without a history of syphilis he was very loth to make a differential diagnosis between the two." ("A Hyperkeratosis of the Sole of the Foot—Possibly of Specific Origin," *Journal of Cutaneous Diseases Including Syphilis* 24:12 [1906], 576).

54. Edward L. Keyes, *The Surgical Diseases of the Genito-Urinary Organs Including Syphilis* (New York: Appleton, 1896), 535; Abner Post, "Errors in the Diagnosis of Syphilis," *Boston Medical and Surgical Journal*, February 13, 1902, 172.

55. The patient case files for this hospital are contained in record group 112, Office of the Surgeon General (Army), Letterman General Hospital, Clinical Records, San Francisco, 1898–1913. For the specific records cited, see Mark Cook, box 1; Joseph Hammond, box 167; John Portwood, box 167; and Joseph K. Latvia, box 276.

56. John Portwood, box 167, Letterman General Hospital.

57. Jason Race, box 167, Letterman General Hospital.

58. Henry O'Kinke, box 167, Letterman General Hospital.

59. *Report of the Surgeon-General* (Washington, DC: Government Printing Office, 1909), 188.

60. "Hospital," *New International Encyclopedia*, vol. 11 (New York: Dodd, Mead, 1915), 503.

61. Herbert G. Aldenbruck, box 1; Bernhard Goldstein, box 20; Thomas Hemstead, box 24. See also George Cummings, box 12.

62. For a similar case, see Clinton Payne, box 43.

63. Gray, "The Diagnosis of One Form of Intra-Cranial Syphilis," 31.

64. For another example of this, see Fay Boardman, box 5.

65. For a similar case, see Alexander Hallbrook, box 22.

66. A typical example here was that of Stannish Kondeck, a soldier admitted to the Letterman Hospital on February 12, 1912, on account of ambulatory difficulties related to his flat feet. Despite having no evidence of a venereal infection, doctors immediately ordered a Wasserman test, which came back negative. For more on this, see William Holitz and Stannish Kondeck, box 275, Letterman Hospital. For similar cases, see Patrick McDonnell, box 275; Luther Felker, box 275, Robert Evans, box 275; David McNab, box 275; Thomas McFadden, box 276; James Martin, box 276; and William Gillen, box 277, Letterman Hospital.

67. When Henry J. Rausch entered the Letterman Hospital on March 15, 1912, he informed the ward surgeon that he had never had a venereal disease, and the surgeon's physical examination revealed no evidence of venereal disease, but after Rausch's Wassermann results came back positive, he was placed on a course of antisyphilitic treatment. For the details of this case, see Henry J. Rausch, box 277, Letterman Hospital. For simi-

lar examples, see Royal Glenister, box 277; and James Nehear, box 277, Letterman Hospital.

68. For a notable example of this, see the case of James P. Size, box 277, Letterman Hospital. For another case along these lines, see William H. Muster, box 277, Letterman Hospital.

69. For an example of the former, see Samuel Pepper, box 43.

70. For evidence of these interactions, see George Harrington, box 17.

71. William Deadrick, "The Diagnosis of Syphilitic Aortitis," *Journal of the Arkansas Medical Society* 19:6 (1922): 110.

72. W. T. Wooton, "A Consideration of the Non-Venereal Infected Prostate," *Journal of the Arkansas Medical Society* 19:12 (1923): 234; Paul Z. Browne, "Diagnosis of the Inflammation of the Male Urethra," *Journal of the Arkansas Medical Society* 28:6 (1931): 106. Alternatively, hospital medical men's nonlaboratory modes of diagnosis may have simply reflected standard practice within the United States military, as it seems that the Wassermann failed to make significant inroads among the medical officers employed within the various branches of the armed forces. For evidence of this, see L. Mervin Maus, "Venereal Diseases in the United States Army—Their Prevention and Treatment," *Military Surgeon* 27:2 (1910): 130–48; and Harold Wellington, "The Masquerader, Syphilis—Some Statistics from Hospital Practice," *Military Surgeon* 28:6 (1911): 649–52.

73. O. C. Butler, "The Importance of an Early Diagnosis of Syphilis," *Journal of the Arkansas Medical Society* 17:10 (1921): 195.

74. For more on this, see Löwy, "Testing for a Sexually Transmissible Disease," 74–92.

75. For a similar example, see Jesse McKinney, box 36.

Chapter 4 · The Hot Springs VD Clinic

1. H. S. Cumming to Charles M. Pearce, January 29, 1936, record group 90, General Records of the Venereal Disease (VD) Division, 1918–36, Records of the Public Health Service, 1912–68, National Archives, College Park, MD.

2. Available federal census information indicates that in 1930, Ishcomer was married and had a least one son. Her husband appears to have been a mill hand, but no occupation is listed for her. Exactly which of her conditions triggered resentment by clinic doctors is not clear.

3. For a brief overview of the Hot Springs VD clinic, see Edwina Walls, "Hot Springs Waters and the Treatment of Venereal Diseases: The U.S. Public Health Service Clinic and Camp Garraday," *Journal of the Arkansas Medical Society* 91:9 (1995): 430–37.

4. Allan Brandt, *No Magic Bullet: A Social History of Venereal Disease in the United States since 1880* (New York: Oxford University Press, 1987), 5.

5. Suzanne Poirier, *Chicago's War on Syphilis, 1937–40: The Times, "the Trib," and the Clap Doctor* (Urbana: University of Illinois Press, 1995), 153.

6. Poirier, *Chicago's War on Syphilis*, 71.

7. Oliver C. Wenger, "The Indigent, Transient Problem and Its Relation to Public Health," Oliver C. Wenger Papers, University of Arkansas for Medical Sciences Archives.

8. Olive C. Wenger, "The Need for Social Hygiene," Wenger Papers.

9. For more on this, see Paul A. Lombardo and Gregory M. Dorr, "Eugenics, Medical Education, and the Public Health Service: Another Perspective on the Tuskegee Syphilis

Experiment," *Bulletin of the History of Medicine* 80:2 (2006): 313; and Christopher Crenner, "The Tuskegee Syphilis Study and the Scientific Concept of Racial Nervous Resistance," *Journal of the History of Medicine and Allied Sciences* 67:2 (2012): 244–80.

10. See Nancy K. Bristow, *Making Men Moral: Social Engineering during the Great War* (New York: New York University Press, 1996). See also Alexandra M. Lord, "Models of Masculinity: Sex Education, the United States Public Health Service, and the YMCA, 1919–24," *Journal of the History of Medicine and Allied Sciences* 58:2 (2003): 123–52.

11. For the Chamberlain-Kahn Act, see Alexandra M. Lord, "Naturally Clean and Wholesome: Women, Sex Education, and the United States Public Health Service, 1918–1928," *Social History of Medicine* 17:3 (2004): 423–41.

12. Victor C. Vaughan, "Protection of American Army against Social Diseases by More Rigid Health Laws," *Pennsylvania Medical Journal* 22:1 (1918): 26. According to Vaughan, the venereal disease rate at Camp Pike was 568.7 per 1,000 soldiers. See also "Disease Conditions among Troops in the United States: Extracts from Telegraphic Reports Received in the Office of the Surgeon-General for the Week Ending October 19, 1917," *Journal of the American Medical Association* 69:18 (1917): 1535–36; and "Venereal Disease and Birth Control," *Journal of the Switchmen's Union* 20:11 (1918): 756.

13. For evidence of this, see the letters of Archie A. Cowles, a syphilitic health seeker who first traveled to Hot Springs in 1905. In a letter dated December 10, 1905, Cowles wrote that "many of the women here seem to be on the courtesan order." "Of course, it would not do to call them prostitutes," Cowles added, "for they are aristocrats in their profession." For Cowles's correspondence, see the Archie A. Cowles Papers, which can be found at the Garland Historical Society.

14. "Commissioners Issue Order to the City Manager to Close the Houses of Immorality, Which Goes into Effect at Once," *Hot Springs Sentinel-Record*, August 2, 1918. Local businessmen and religious leaders rejected the association the military made between Camp Pike's high venereal disease rate and the "terrible conditions" in Hot Springs. See "Ministerial Men to Discuss Morals: Report from Washington of Bad Conditions Here Stirs Some Enthusiasts," *Hot Springs Sentinel-Record*, August 9, 1918, and "The Moral Condition," *Hot Springs Sentinel-Record*, August 10, 1918.

15. Audrey Wenger McCully, "The United States Public Health Service Venereal Disease Clinic and Government Free Bathhouse, 1919–1936," Wenger Papers.

16. "Proceedings of the Minnesota Academy of Medicine," *Minnesota Medicine* 5:1 (1922): 61.

17. *First Deficiency Appropriation Bill, 1921: Hearings before Subcommittee of House Committee on Appropriations,* 66th Congress, 3rd Session (Washington, DC: Government Printing Office, 1921), 588.

18. *First Deficiency Appropriation Bill, 1921,* 560, 568.

19. This last point holds for all of the public health campaigns undertaken in the early twentieth-century US South. In the case of Hot Springs, the city was seen as a center of quackery and, in particular, of the country's VD patent medicine industry. See *Excluding Advertisements of Cures for Venereal Diseases from the Mails: Hearings before the Committee on the Post Office and Post Roads of the House of Representatives,* 66th Congress, 1st Session (Washington, DC: Government Printing Office, 1921).

20. During the war, Wenger—a native of St. Louis—served in the Medical Corps of the Missouri National Guard and then as a member of Sanitary Squad 18, stationed in

Camp Mills, New York, where he focused his efforts on "venereal disease prophylaxis." After the war, Wenger sought and obtained appointment as a "regional consultant" in the PHS, where he assisted in the nationwide venereal disease survey (1919–20) (McCully, "The United States Public Health Service Venereal Disease Clinic and Government Free Bathhouse").

21. For more on Wenger's life, see McCully, "The United States Public Health Service Venereal Disease Clinic and Government Free Bathhouse."

22. Susan Reverby, *Examining Tuskegee: The Infamous Syphilis Study and Its Legacy* (Chapel Hill: University of North Carolina Press, 2009), 141.

23. Oliver C. Wenger to C. C. Pierce, March 16, 1921, National Park Service (NPS) Archives, Hot Springs, AR.

24. Oliver C. Wenger, "Instructions" (1921), Wenger Papers.

25. Oliver C. Wenger to Dr. White, January 13, 1925, VD Division Records.

26. For more on this, see a pamphlet prepared by the PHS entitled *Instructions to Medical Officers in Charge of the Control of Venereal Diseases* (Washington, DC: Government Printing Office, 1918).

27. Oliver C. Wenger to W. B. Grayson, November 19, 1935, VD Division Records.

28. Wenger to Grayson, November 19, 1935.

29. Oliver C. Wenger to J. W. Brown, November 12, 1935, VD Division Records.

30. Wenger, "Instructions."

31. McCully, "The United States Public Health Service Venereal Disease Clinic and Government Free Bathhouse."

32. Oliver C. Wenger, "The United States Public Health Service Clinic at Hot Springs National Park, Arkansas," Wenger Papers.

33. Oliver C. Wenger, "A Comparative Study of the Amount of Money Each Applicant Declared under Oath at the U.S. Government Bath House for the Years 1931–32," Wenger Papers.

34. Oliver C. Wenger, "United States Conducts Clinic for Venereal Diseases," *Nation's Health* 8:2 (1926): 103; McCully, "The United States Public Health Service Venereal Disease Clinic and Government Free Bathhouse."

35. McCully, "The United States Public Health Service Venereal Disease Clinic and Government Free Bathhouse."

36. Virgil Oren Adams to Franklin D. Roosevelt, September 27, 1934, VD Division Records. Part of Adams's story also derives from a letter he sent to Captain Geoffrey (an officer at the Hot Springs clinic) on October 9, 1934, VD Division Records).

37. Oliver C. Wenger to the surgeon general, October 18, 1934, VD Division Records.

38. For evidence of this, consider the case of James Gordon. A Michigan man, in 1926 Gordon wrote the PHS (August 17, 1926, VD Division Records) asking for help in getting to Hot Springs. "I have tried [sic] all kinds of medicines, which you know that it [sic] takes money." From a book he had read, Gordon surmised that "there is not mutch [sic] chance for a poor man there," but still he pleaded. Hot Springs was "the last chance I have got—I have every thing [sic] else until my money is gone."

39. Wenger, "The Need for Social Hygiene."

40. For more on America's fertility transition, see J. David Hacker, "Rethinking the 'Early' Decline of Marital Fertility in the United States," *Demography* 40:4 (2003): 605–20.

41. Abraham L. Wolbarst, "The Venereal Diseases: A Menace to the National Welfare," *Medical Review* 62:10 (1910): 373.

42. For more on this, see Reverby, *Examining Tuskegee*, 139–44.

43. McCully, "The United States Public Health Service Venereal Disease Clinic and Government Free Bathhouse."

44. J. R. Waugh and Elizabeth Milovich, "Severe Reactions to Arsphenamine among 3,050 Previously Untreated Patients," *Journal of Venereal Disease Information* 21:12 (1940): 391. The Hot Springs clinic, it bears noting, was far from the only site where Salvarsan was administered experimentally. In the medical literature of the time, many physicians reported success with an accelerated treatment regimen, and some recommended giving as many as three doses in a twenty-four hour period. One advocate advised colleagues to "give the largest possible amount of salvarsan in the shortest possible time" (Faxton E. Gardner, "The Treatment of Syphilis," *Medical Times* 45:4 [1917]: 63). For other accounts of the intensive and continuous treatment of syphilis with Salvarsan, see Frederick W. Smith, "The Modern Diagnosis and Treatment of Syphilis," *Medical Record*, February 3, 1917, 186–91; B. C. Corbus, "Prophylaxis in Cerebrospinal Syphilis," *Journal of the American Medical Association* 69:25 (1917): 2087–89; and Carlyle N. Haines, "Salvarsan in Syphilis," *Pennsylvania Medical Journal* 24:11 (1921): 839–41.

45. Oliver C. Wenger and Lida J. Usilton, "Notes on the Syphilis Clinic, United States Public Health Service, Hot Springs, Arkansas," *Journal of Venereal Disease Information* 15:6 (1934): 210. It is impossible to verify these morbidity and mortality figures, as the clinic operated free from federal oversight. Because of this and also because of the clinic's generally poor record-keeping practices, the number of "adverse reactions" may have been higher than what Wenger reported. For more on the latter problem, see C. H. Waring to the surgeon general, January 23, 1923, VD Division Records.

46. Waugh and Milosivic's 1940 study "Severe Reactions to Arsphenamine among 3,050 Previously Untreated Patients" notes that clinic personnel revealed that nearly 2.5 patients per 1,000 experienced "severe reactions" to Salvarsan—a rate higher than the 1.99 per 1,000 reported by the Cooperative Clinical Group's studies of syphilis.

47. Wenger and Usilton, "Notes on the Syphilis Clinic, United States Public Health Service, Hot Springs, Arkansas," 209. For further evidence of serious medical complications following on the clinic's intensive plan of syphilis treatment, see George E. Tarkington, "Value of Liver Function Test in Arsenical Therapy," *Journal of Venereal Disease Information* 7:1 (1926): 24–25. For details of a specific injury, see Paul S. Carley, "Infarction of Buttock from Intra-Muscular Injections of Mercury Benzoate," *Journal of Venereal Disease Information* 17:10 (1936): 281–83. It bears noting here that during the 1920s and 1930s, the idea of informed consent had not become a universally recognized principle within medical ethics. Because of this, scientific investigators were not required to obtain patient permission before proceeding with experiments. Those housed within custodial institutions (public hospitals and clinics, asylums, prisons, orphanages etc.) were especially targeted for human subjects research, a practice often justified on the grounds that that they owed society a debt in exchange for the free treatment they received. For more on this, see Susan Lederer, *Subjected to Science: Human Experimentation in America before the Second World War* (Baltimore, MD: Johns Hopkins University Press, 1997).

48. For the details of LaPrade's case, see G. L. Collins to the surgeon general, October 11, 1932, VD Division Records.

49. Forrest D. LaPrade to Wright Patman, June 10, 1930, VD Division Records.

50. For more on this study, see J. R. Waugh, "Treatment of Chronic Endocervicitis of Gonorrheal Origin by Surgical Diathermy," *Journal of Venereal Disease Information* 14:11 (1933): 277–82.

51. M. J. White, "Next Steps in the Field of VD Control from the Standpoint of the United States Public Health Service," *Journal of Venereal Disease Information* 7:1 (1926): 173.

52. "Meeting of the Advisory Committee to the Division of Venereal Diseases, United States Public Health Service, May 16, 1927," *Journal of Venereal Disease Information* 8:8 (1927): 303.

53. C. H. Waring to the surgeon general, January 23, 1923. Waring requested that the clinic's administrative staff be augmented, but this request appears not to have been granted.

54. Waugh and Milovich, "Severe Reactions to Arsphenamine among 3,050 Previously Untreated Patients," 390.

55. Oliver C. Wenger to R. A. Vonderlehr, May 25, 1936, Wenger Papers.

56. T. J. Bauer and H. C. Cecil, "The Treatment of the Severe Complications of Gonorrhea with Hyperpyrexia Produced by the Kettering Hypetherm," *Journal of Venereal Disease Information* 19:8 (1938): 245.

57. Bauer and Cecil, "The Treatment of the Severe Complications of Gonorrhea with Hyperpyrexia Produced by the Kettering Hypetherm," 245–50.

58. Wenger, "The Need for Social Hygiene"; Oliver C. Wenger, *Annual Report for 1923*, Wenger Papers.

59. "Hot Springs Threatened with Loss of Patronage: Health Resort Must Eliminate Red-Light District," *Social Hygiene Bulletin* 8:1 (1921): 8.

60. L. Blance Young to Oliver C. Wenger, February 8, 1932, Wenger Papers.

61. Oliver C. Wenger to David Robinson, April 18, 1921, Wenger Papers.

62. Information on brothel closures comes from my own analysis of Hot Springs police dockets between 1920 and 1923. These documents can be found in the Garland County Historical Society Archives, Hot Springs, AR. In 1918, before the initial crackdown on prostitution, sex workers accounted for almost one-fifth of all criminal arrests in the city.

63. *First Deficiency Appropriation Bill, 1921*, 568.

64. "Hard Sledding for Bankrupt City," *Yearbook of the City Managers' Association* 6 (1920): 85–86.

65. Oliver C. Wenger, "The Transient-Indigent-Medical Problem at Hot Springs National Park, Arkansas," Wenger Papers.

66. Ray Hanley, *A Place Apart: A Pictorial History of Hot Springs, Arkansas* (Fayetteville: University of Arkansas Press, 2011), 81; Webb Waldron, "Sin Takes a Holiday," March 31, 1934, 23.

67. James T. Jelks, "Annual Address of the President on the Prevention of Venereal Diseases," *Journal of the Arkansas Medical Society* 3:12 (1893): 539.

68. G. O. Hebert, "Venereal Prophylaxis," *Journal of the Arkansas Medical Society* 6:4 (1909): 115.

69. Wenger, "The Transient-Indigent-Medical Problem at Hot Springs National Park, Arkansas."

70. Wenger, *Annual Report for 1923*.

71. Oliver C. Wenger, "History of United States Public Health Clinic, Hot Springs, Arkansas," Wenger Papers.

72. "Any person who engages in travel," Wenger maintained, "may be the carrier of a communicable disease." "Every health officer knows," he reminded his superiors, "of instances, when, from one single source, hundreds and thousands of new cases have developed" ("The Indigent, Transient Problem and Its Relation to Public Health").

73. Wenger, "The Indigent, Transient Problem and Its Relation to Public Health." In connection with Wenger's apparent acceptance of prostitution in Hot Springs, it is interesting to note that while overseeing a VD control program in Puerto Rico during the Second World War, the PHS official was privately reprimanded for proposing "methods of registration and identification of prostitutes which seem quite out of line" with the federal government's official policy of repression. For more on this see, Thomas Parran to Oliver C. Wenger, March 23, 1942, series 1, box 5, Thomas Parran Papers, University of Pittsburgh.

74. Oliver C. Wenger to Thomas Parran, October 23, 1926, series 1, box 5, Thomas Parran Papers, University of Pittsburgh; Oliver C. Wenger to Dr. White, January 13, 1925, VD Division Records.

75. Wenger to White, January 13, 1925.

76. Wenger, "The Transient-Indigent-Medical Problem at Hot Springs National Park, Arkansas."

77. Wenger, "The Transient-Indigent-Medical Problem at Hot Springs National Park, Arkansas."

78. Oliver C. Wenger, "Summary Statistical Data," Wenger Papers.

79. Oliver C. Wenger, "An Analysis of 10,000 Cases of Syphilis," Wenger Papers.

80. See Waugh and Milovich, "Severe Reactions to Arsphenamine among 3,050 Previously Untreated Patients," 390. For further evidence of the comparatively unfavorable therapeutic outcomes the clinic's black patients met with, see J. R. Waugh and W. Burns Jones, "Genito-Urinary Survey of 1,625 Male Patients, United States Public Health Service Venereal Disease Clinic, Hot Springs, Ark.," *Journal of Venereal Disease Information* 13:1 (1932): 9.

81. Walter Martin to Oliver C. Wenger, March 2, 1928, VD Division Records.

82. Between 1922 and 1932, the number of African American visitors listed in the "unskilled labor" category was "nearly twice as high" as the comparable figure for whites (Wenger, "An Analysis of 10,000 Cases of Syphilis").

83. Wenger, "An Analysis of 10,000 Cases of Syphilis."

84. A. W. Hunton, "The American Carlsbad," *Voice of the Negro* 3:5 (1906): 331; C. Melnotte Wade, "Hot Springs—Its People," *Colored American Magazine* 10:1 (1906):13; Wenger, "The United States Public Health Service Clinic at Hot Springs National Park, Arkansas"; Oliver C. Wenger to the surgeon general, July 27, 1934, VD Division Records.

85. Wenger to Parran, October 23, 1926, Thomas Parran Papers.

86. Oliver C. Wenger to the surgeon general, July 20, 1925, VD Division Records.

87. For this, see Paul Carley, "Infection with Syphilis Masked by Gonorrhea," *Journal of Venereal Disease Information* 18:2 (1937): 23.

88. "Officer Uses 'Gestapo' Methods: Texarkanians Terrorized, Business Houses Molested," *Arkansas State Press*, July 25, 1941, 1, 6.

89. "Officer Uses 'Gestapo' Methods."

90. "Hot Springs Judge Wroth over 'Dumping' of Indigent Diseased Transients in City," Wenger Papers; Wenger, "The Transient-Indigent-Medical Problem at Hot Springs National Park, Arkansas; Wenger to the surgeon general, July 27, 1934.

91. Wenger, "United States Conducts Clinic for Venereal Diseases," 103.

92. For more on this, see Michael Grey, *New Deal Medicine: The Rural Health Programs of the Farm Security Administration* (Baltimore, MD: Johns Hopkins University Press, 2002).

93. Grey, *New Deal Medicine*, 33.

94. For more on this, see Erin Wuebker, "Taking the Venereal out of Venereal Disease: The Public Health Campaign against Syphilis, 1934–34" (PhD diss., City University of New York, 2015).

95. Wuebker, "Taking the Venereal out of Venereal Disease," 152.

96. Oliver C. Wenger, "A Plan for the Consolidation of All Medical Measures for Transient Relief in Hot Springs, Arkansas" (September 5, 1935), NPS Archives.

97. Wenger, "A Plan for the Consolidation of All Medical Measures for Transient Relief in Hot Springs, Arkansas"; Wenger, "The Indigent, Transient Problem and Its Relation to Public Health."

98. Wenger, "The Indigent, Transient Problem and Its Relation to Public Health," emphasis added.

99. Grey, *New Deal Medicine*, 35.

100. For more on these camps, see Grey, *New Deal Medicine*, 85–93.

101. Oliver C. Wenger to Taliaferro Clark, August 29, 1931, NPS Archives.

102. Oliver C. Wenger, "The Transient-Indigent-Medical Program," Wenger Papers.

103. Wenger, "The Transient-Indigent-Medical Problem at Hot Springs National Park, Arkansas."

104. R. O. Brunk, "Some Interesting Facts," Wenger Papers.

105. Oliver C. Wenger to R.A. Vonderlehr, January 10, 1934, NPS Archives.

106. Wenger, "The United States Public Health Service Clinic at Hot Springs National Park, Arkansas."

107. Antoinette Cannon, "Hot Springs Transient Program" (1935), Wenger Papers.

108. McCully, "The United States Public Health Service Venereal Disease Clinic and Government Free Bathhouse."

109. For evidence of this, see VD Division Records.

110. Wenger to the surgeon general, July 27, 1934.

111. Brunk, "Some Interesting Facts"; "Hot Springs Judge Wroth over 'Dumping' of Indigent Diseased Transients in City."

112. "Hot Springs Judge Wroth over 'Dumping' of Indigent Diseased Transients in City."

113. Wenger, "A Plan for the Consolidation of All Medical Measures for Transient Relief in Hot Springs, Arkansas," NPS Archives.

114. "Council Approves New Transient Plan," Wenger Papers.

115. Lucile Mulhall to Oliver C. Wenger, February 11, 1935, Wenger Papers.

116. Mulhall to Wenger, February 11, 1935; Cannon, "Hot Springs Transient Program."

117. R. C. Brunk, "Is a Camp Practicable for the Transients at the Hot Springs Division Arkansas Transient Bureau?" (July 26, 1934), RG 69.3.3, Records of the Transient Division, National Archives.

118. H. W. Gilmore to W. R. Dyess, July 9, 1934, Records of the Transient Division.

119. Brunk, "Is a Camp Practicable for the Transients at the Hot Springs Division Arkansas Transient Bureau?"

120. Gilmore to Dyess, July 9, 1934

121. Oliver C. Wenger, "Proposed Plan for Adequate Medical Service for Transients at Hot Springs National Park, Arkansas," Records of Transient Division; Cannon, "Hot Springs Transient Program."

122. Gilmore to Dyess, July 9, 1934.

123. Wenger, "A Plan for the Consolidation of All Medical Measures for Transient Relief in Hot Springs, Arkansas."

124. This description was provided by Mary D. Hudgins, a native Arkansan who worked with the Federal Writers' Project during the Great Depression. For more information, see "Emma Sanderson" in *Slave Narratives: A Folk History of Slavery in the United States from Interviews with Former Slaves*, vol. 2, *Arkansas*, pt. 6, Quinn-Tuttle (Washington, DC: Government Printing Office, 1941), 118.

125. Wenger, "A Plan for the Consolidation of All Medical Measures for Transient Relief in Hot Springs, Arkansas."

126. Wenger, "The United States Public Health Service Clinic at Hot Springs National Park, Arkansas."

127. Wuebker, "Taking the Venereal out of Venereal Disease," 195–96, 197.

128. *A Review of Work Relief Activities in Arkansas* (Little Rock: Arkansas State Emergency Relief Administration, 1935), 106.

129. *A Review of Work Relief Activities in Arkansas*, 106.

130. Wenger, "A Plan for the Consolidation of All Medical Measures for Transient Relief in Hot Springs, Arkansas."

131. As one local authority put it, developments of the early 1930s had given the health resort's more wealthy visitors the impression that "the transients being treated here were so numerous that [they] would overrun everything," and on account of this, the city had become "undesirable for pay patients" (Thomas J. Allen to Arno B. Cammerer, July 23, 1934, NPS Archives).

132. John J. McShane to all local health authorities, March 10, 1936, VD Division Records.

133. "Venereal Disease Control," *Arkansas Health Bulletin* 1:3 (1944): 6–9.

Chapter 5 · From Hygiene to Hydrotherapy

1. Edward H. Martin to William P. Parks, March 10, 1921, National Park Service (NPS) Archives, Hot Springs, Arkansas.

2. William P. Parks to Stephen H. Mather, April 2, 1921, NPS Archives.

3. Edward H. Martin to William P. Parks, March 10, 1921, NPS Archives.

4. Edward H. Martin to Stephen H. Mather, March 13, 1921, NPS Archives.

5. "Report of the Medical Director of the Hot Springs Reservation, Arkansas," *Reports of the Department of the Interior for the Fiscal Year That Ended June 30, 1911* (Washington, DC: Government Printing Office, 1912), 762.

6. W. T. Wooton, "The Adequate Treatment of Syphilis," *Medical Record*, July 8, 1911, 95.

7. Admitting as much, just as Edward Martin downsized his operations, Oliver Wenger in a letter to David Robinson on March 24, 1921, wrote of how "the local profession are be-

ginning to feel the effects of our work" (record group 90, General Records of the Venereal Disease [VD] Division, 1918–36, Records of the Public Health Service, 1912–68, National Archives, College Park, MD).

8. William S. Ehrich, "Treatment of Syphilis," *Journal of the Indiana State Medical Association* 6:11 (1913): 348.

9. Edward H. Martin, "The Arkansas Hot Springs Baths," *Southern Medical Journal* 9:3 (1916): 212.

10. For an overview of medical holism in the early twentieth century, see Christopher Lawrence and George Weisz, eds., *Greater than the Parts: Holism in Western Biomedicine, 1920–1950* (New York: Oxford University Press, 1998).

11. Christopher Lawrence and George Weisz, "Medical Holism: The Context," in *Greater than the Parts*, 1–22.

12. Sarah W. Tracy, "An Evolving Science of Man: The Transformation and Demise of American Constitutional Medicine, 1920–1950," in *Greater than the Parts*, 163.

13. For more on this, see Matthew Frye Jacobson, *The Barbarian Virtues: The United States Encounters Foreign Peoples at Home and Abroad, 1876–1917* (New York: Hill and Wang, 2000).

14. As one recent study has noted, instead of disappearing, the Hippocratic "Airs, Waters, and Places" tradition "has been redeployed with regularity in a range of new contexts, and to diverse ends over the past century" (Alison Bashford and Sarah W. Tracey, "Modern Airs, Waters, and Places," *Bulletin of the History of Medicine* 86:4 [2012]: 511).

15. Jacobson, *Barbarian Virtues*.

16. For an account of American public health efforts in the Philippines, see Warwick Anderson, *Colonial Pathologies: American Tropical Medicine, Race, and Hygiene in the Philippines* (Durham, NC: Duke University Press, 2006).

17. Notably, this was true of other Western imperial powers as well. The French, for one, made extensive use of hydrotherapy throughout their colonies. As one recent history of the subject concludes, their promotion and use owed entirely to fears of white fragility in the tropics. See Eric T. Jennings, *Curing the Colonizers: Hydrotherapy, Climatology, and French Colonial Spas* (Durham, NC: Duke University Press, 2006).

18. *Report of the Commissioner of Public Health for the Philippine Islands, for the Year Ended September 1, 1903* (Washington, DC: Government Printing Office, 1903), 217.

19. George F. Becker, *Report on the Geology of the Philippine Islands* (Washington, DC: Government Printing Office, 1901), 48.

20. M. Saderra Maso, *Volcanoes and Seismic Centers of the Philippine Archipelago*, vol. 3 of *Census of the Philippine Islands* (Washington, DC: Government Printing Office, 1904), 18.

21. "The Climate of Baguio, Island of Luzon," *Bulletin of the American Geographical Society of New York* 35:2 (1903): 195.

22. "The Climate of Baguio, Island of Luzon," 195.

23. *What Has Been Done in the Philippines: A Record of Practical Accomplishments under Civil Government* (Washington, DC: Government Printing Office, 1904), 38–39.

24. *What Has Been Done in the Philippines*, 38.

25. *Agriculture, Social, and Industrial Statistics*, vol. 4 of *Census of the Philippine Islands* (Washington, DC: Government Printing Office, 1905), 600.

26. *Annual Report of the Bureau of Health* (Manila: Bureau of Printing, 1905), 56.

27. *Description of the Philippines*, pt. 1 (Manila: Bureau of Public Printing, 1903), 54.

28. Theodore W. Noyes, *Oriental America and Its Problems* (Washington, DC: Judd and Detweiler, 1903), 101.

29. For more on this phenomenon, see Bashford and Tracey, "Modern Airs, Waters, and Places," 495–514.

30. Michael Osborne and Richard S. Fogarty, "Medical Climatology in France: The Persistence of Neo-Hippocratic Ideas in the First Half of the Twentieth Century," *Bulletin of the History of Medicine* 86:4 (2012): 543–63.

31. James C. Minor, "The Health and Wealth of Benguet Province, P.I." *Journal of the American Medical Association* 35:15 (1900): 948.

32. Minor, "The Health and Wealth of Benguet Province, P.I.," 949.

33. *Annual Report of the Bureau of Health*, 56; Frederic H. Sawyer, *The Inhabitants of the Philippines* (New York: Charles Scribner's Sons, 1900), 157.

34. *Description of the Philippines.* 53.

35. Louis M. Maus, "Military Sanitary Problems in the Philippine Islands," *Military Surgeon* 24:1 (1909): 31.

36. "The American Soldier and Venereal Diseases," *Medical Review*, August 26, 1899, 149.

37. "Due to the fact that venereal cases come here from Manila for treatment," one report on Los Baños explained, "there is a large percentage of venereal disease among the native women. The cause is obvious." This report went on to state that "over 80 percent" of patients treated at Los Baños were suffering from syphilis or gonorrhea. See *Report of the Commissioner of Public Health for the Philippine Islands, for the Year Ended September 1, 1903*, 217.

38. James C. Minor, "Renal Insufficiency in the Tropics," *Journal of the American Medical Association* 39:2 (1902): 1254–56; *Affairs in the Philippine Islands; Hearings before the Committee on the Philippines of the United States Senate, April 10, 1902* (Washington, DC: Government Printing Office, 1902), 1639.

39. Minor, "Renal Insufficiency in the Tropics," 1254–56.

40. James C. Minor, "Philippines Customs and Habits," *Journal of the American Medical Society* 37:24 (1901): 1702.

41. Minor, "The Health and Wealth of Benguet Province, P.I.," 949.

42. Minor, "Philippines Health and Customs," 1702–3.

43. See Anthony Rotundo, *American Manhood: Transformations in Masculinity from the Revolution to the Modern Era* (New York: Basic Books, 1994).

44. For scholarly discussions of these trends, see Elliot J. Gorn, *The Manly Art: Bare-Knuckle Prize Fighting in America* (Ithaca, NY: Cornell University Press, 2010).

45. For more on the consumption of Indian patent medicines, see John Rosenberg, "Barbarian Virtues in a Bottle: Patent Indian Medicines and the Commodification of Primitivism in the United States, 1870–1900," *Gender and History* 24:2 (2012): 368–88. See also Laura Briggs, "The Race of Hysteria: 'Overcivilization' and the 'Savage' Woman in Late Nineteenth-Century Obstetrics and Gynecology," *American Quarterly* 52:2 (2000): 246–73.

46. James. C. Minor, "Water, the Main Factor in the Treatment of Disease," *Dietetic and Hygienic Gazette* 27:2 (1912): 92.

47. Minor, "Water, the Main Factor in the Treatment of Disease," 93.

48. Minor, "Water, the Main Factor in the Prevention of Disease," 83.

49. Minor, "Water, the Main Factor in the Prevention of Disease.," 83.

50. Edward H. Martin, "A Drugless Clinic," *Memphis Medical Monthly* 28:4 (1908): 197.

51. William O. Forbes, "Cases Illustrating the Dangers of Salvarsan and Kindred Preparations in the Treatment of Syphilis," *Journal of the American Institute of Homeopathy* 8:5 (1915): 532.

52. Loyd Thompson, *Syphilis* (Philadelphia: Lea and Febiger, 1917), 211.

53. Loyd Thompson, "Hydrotherapy in Syphilis," *American Journal of Physical Therapy* 8:11 (1931): 216.

54. Thompson, "Hydrotherapy in Syphilis," 216.

55. Thomas Black and W. M. Blackshare, "Hydrotherapy in the Treatment of Syphilis," *Tri-State Medical Journal* 2:7 (1930): 336.

56. E. A. Purdum, "The Thermal Baths in the Treatment of Syphilis," *Journal of the Arkansas Medical Society* 27:7 (1930): 138.

57. E. A. Purdum, "Further Observations Regarding Heat Therapy in the Treatment of Syphilis," *Tri-State Medical Journal* 3:11 (1931): 665.

58. Patricia Ward Spain, "The American Reception of Salvarsan," *Journal of the History of Medicine and Allied Sciences* 36:1 (1981): 44–62.

59. Abner H. Cook, "The Diagnostic Value of the Reaction Following the Intravenous Injection of Salvarsan, with a Few Remarks upon the Therapeutic Value of the Drug," *Journal of the Arkansas Medical Society* 9:5 (1912): 118–27.

60. Estill D. Holland, "A Report of One Hundred Cases of Syphilis Treated with Salvarsan," *Medical Herald* 30:6 (1911): 251.

61. A. J. Whitworth and J. M. Byrd, *The Hot Springs Specialist* (Memphis: S. C. Toof, 1913), 164.

62. Howard P. Collings, "Treatment of Syphilis with 'Salvarsan,'" *Journal of the Arkansas Medical Society* 8:3 (1911): 85.

63. For an example of this, see Charles W. Hitchcock, "The Treatment of Luetic Diseases of the Nervous System," *Journal of the Michigan State Medical Society* 13:11 (1914): 647.

64. Even with the emergence of Salvarsan, many doctors counted the healers of Hot Springs among the nation's foremost experts in venereology. For evidence of this, see Granville MacGowan, "The Treatment of Syphilis," *Urologic and Cutaneous Review* 20:7 (1916): 361–69.

65. H. J. Farbach, "Further Results with the Use of Salvarsanized Serum," *Kentucky Medical Journal* 13:7 (1915): 267.

66. J. Garland Sherrill, "Tertiary Syphilis: Report of Three Cases," *Kentucky Medical Journal* 19:8 (1921): 507.

67. Forbes, "Cases Illustrating the Dangers of Salvarsan and Kindred Preparations in the Treatment of Syphilis," 530.

68. Collings, "Treatment of Syphilis with 'Salvarsan.'" Southern physicians in particular noted how Salvarsan's spread obviated the need to send their patients to Hot Springs; see B. N. Dunvant, "Report of 7 Cases of Syphilis Treated with '606,'" *Memphis Medical Monthly* 31:6 (1911): 281–86.

69. Henry H. Morton, *Genitourinary Diseases and Syphilis* (Philadelphia: F. A. Davis, 1912), 550, 760. See also Wooton, "The Adequate Treatment of Syphilis," 95.

70. Edward H. Martin, "Discussion on Papers by Drs. Dyer and Thompson," *Southern Medical Journal* 9:2 (1916): 138–39. The cited remarks were given by Martin in response to a paper by Loyd Thompson on the public health aspects of syphilis.

71. Oliver C. Wenger, "The Early Days of Hot Springs, Arkansas (1850–1900)," Oliver C. Wenger Papers, University of Arkansas for Medical Sciences Archives.

72. Frederick Forcheimer, *Forcheimer's Therapeusis of Internal Diseases*, vol. 2 (New York: Appleton, 1920), 420.

73. Forcheimer, *Forcheimer's Therapeusis of Internal Diseases*, 420.

74. Woods Hutchinson, "Taking the Waters: The Humbug of Hot Springs," *Everybody's Magazine* 28:2 (1913): 166.

75. Hutchinson, "Taking the Waters," 160.

76. Hutchinson, "Taking the Waters," 160.

77. Wooton, "The Adequate Treatment of Syphilis," 304.

78. Oliver C. Wenger to United States Public Health Service Advisory Board, September 28, 1921, Wenger Papers.

79. Oliver C. Wenger to surgeon general, United States Public Health Service, September 15, 1922, Wenger Papers.

80. C. H. Waring, report to surgeon general on Hot Springs, 1923, Wenger Papers.

81. Oliver C. Wenger to David Robinson, March 24, 1921, VD Division Records.

82. C. C. Pierce, "The Relationship of Local, State, and Federal Agencies in Venereal Disease Control," *Southern Medical Journal* 15:2 (1922): 121–29.

83. Pierce, "The Relationship of Local, State, and Federal Agencies in Venereal Disease Control," 123.

84. Talafierro Clark and Lida J. Usilton, "Trend of Cases of Syphilis under Treatment or Observation in the United States," *Southern Medical Journal* 26:8 (1933): 726.

85. W. T. Wooton, "Family Physician versus Laboratory Diagnosis of Malaria," *Southern Medical Journal* 18:2 (1925): 116.

86. Abner Cook, "The Evolution of Knowledge Pertaining to Syphilis," *Journal of the Arkansas Medical Society* 11:2 (1914): 39.

87. Minor, "Water, the Main Factor in the Prevention of Disease," 89.

88. Scholars estimate that the so-called Spanish flu killed at least twenty million worldwide. For a discussion of the United States' response to the pandemic, see Carol R. Byerly, *Fever of War: The Influenza Epidemic in the U.S. Army during World War I* (New York: New York University Press, 2005).

89. Lawrence and George Weisz, "Medical Holism," 1–14.

90. Michael Hau, "The Holistic Gaze in German Medicine, 1890–1930," *Bulletin of the History of Medicine* 74:3 (2000): 495–524.

91. George Weisz, "Hippocrates, Holism, and Humanism in Interwar France," in *Reinventing Hippocrates*, ed. David Cantor (Burlington, VT: Ashgate, 2002), 268.

92. David Cantor, "The Uses and Meanings of Hippocrates," in *Reinventing Hippocrates*, ed. David Cantor (Burlington, VT: Ashgate, 2002), 13.

93. Osborne and Fogarty, "Medical Climatology in France."

94. Andrew Hull, "Glasgow's 'Sick Society'? James Halliday, Psychosocial Medicine and Medical Holism in Britain, c. 1920–1948," *History of the Human Sciences* 25:5 (2012): 73–90.

95. Sarah W. Tracey, "An Evolving Science of Man: The Transformation and Demise of American Constitutional Medicine, 1920–1950," in *Greater than the Parts*, 163.

96. James T. Jelks, "The Antiquity of Syphilis, and Moses as a Health Officer," *Journal of the American Medical Association* 21:4 (1893): 105.

97. Estill D. Holland, "The Use of Radioactive Waters; with Special Reference to Those at Hot Springs," *American Journal of Clinical Medicine* 19:11 (1912): 1108–9.

98. C. Travis Drennen, "Hydrotherapy," *Journal of the Arkansas Medical Society* 12:3 (1915): 81.

99. Purdum, "The Thermal Baths in the Treatment of Syphilis," 135.

100. For evidence of this, see Mitchell B. Hart, "'They Dedicated Themselves to the Abominable Idol': Ancient Hebrew Sexuality and Modern Medical Diagnosis," *Jewish Social Studies: History, Culture, Society* 21:3 (2016): 72–90.

101. Loyd Thompson, "Some of the Unsolved Problems of Syphilis," *Journal of the Arkansas Medical Society* 17:3 (1930): 50.

102. Purdum, "The Thermal Baths in the Treatment of Syphilis," 135, 137.

103. George M. Eckel, "The Diagnosis of Neuro-Syphilis," *Journal of the Arkansas Medical Society* 19:5 (1920): 82.

104. Thomas N. Black and Jett Scott, "Powders and Potents," *Journal of the Arkansas Medical Society* 18:12 (1937): 215; George M. Eckel, "Cardiac Neuroses," *Journal of the Arkansas Medical Society* 18:7 (1921): 142.

105. Euclid M. Smith, "Underwater Therapy in the Treatment of Chronic Arthritis," *Journal of the Arkansas Medical Society* 32:9 (1936): 138.

106. Black and Scott, "Powders and Potents," 215.

107. Black and Scott, "Powders and Potents," 215–16.

108. Black and Blackshare, "Hydrotherapy," 336.

109. Purdum, "The Thermal Baths in the Treatment of Syphilis," 139.

110. Purdum, "The Thermal Baths in the Treatment of Syphilis," 138.

111. Loyd Thompson, "Some of the Unresolved Problems of Syphilis," 53.

112. Purdum, "The Thermal Baths in the Treatment of Syphilis," 139. The physician who uttered these remarks was C. Travis Drennen.

113. Louis M. Maus, "Hydrology in the Treatment of Diseases, Injuries, and Disorders Incident to Military Service," *Medical Herald* 43:12 (1924): 278.

114. Maus, "Hydrology in the Treatment of Diseases, Injuries, and Disorders Incident to Military Service," 209.

115. Oliver C. Wenger, "A Study of Hydrotherapy in Relation to the Treatment of Syphilis," *Venereal Disease Information* 10:8 (1929): 327.

116. M. R. Richards, "The Hot Baths at Hot Springs," *American Medicine*, n.s., 3:10 (1908): 477.

117. Purdum, "The Thermal Baths in the Treatment of Syphilis," 138.

118. Purdum, "The Thermal Baths in the Treatment of Syphilis," 139. The physician who made this statement was Drennen.

119. Maus, "Hydrology in the Treatment of Diseases," 276.

120. Maus, "Hydrology in the Treatment of Diseases," 276.

121. For one example of this, see "Our Own Carlsbad," *Godey's Magazine* 128:764 (1894): 13–16.

122. Harry M. Hallock, "Some Aspects of Hydrotherapy in the United States," in *Transactions of the Section on Pharmacology and Therapeutics of the American Medical Association* (Chicago: American Medical Association Press, 1913), 147.

123. Purdum, "Further Observations Regarding Heat Therapy in the Treatment of Syphilis," 666.

124. Thomas N. Black and W. M. Blackshare, "Hydrotherapy in the Treatment of Syphilis," *Tri-State Medical Journal* 2:9 (1930): 336.

125. Holland, "The Use of Radioactive Waters," 1109.

126. Bertram B. Boltwood, "On the Radio-Active Properties of the Waters of the Springs on the Hot Springs Reservation, Hot Springs, Arkansas," *American Journal of Science* 20:116 (1905): 128–32.

127. Francis J. Scully, "The Role of Radio Activity of Natural Spring Waters as a Therapeutic Agent," *Journal of the Arkansas Medical Society* 30:11 (1934): 210.

128. Edward H. Martin, "Further Observations on the Physiological Effects of the Waters of the Hot Springs of Arkansas," *New Orleans Medical and Surgical Journal* 60:9 (1908): 731.

129. Holland, "The Use of Radioactive Waters," 1109.

130. Martin, "Further Observations on the Physiological Effects of the Waters of the Hot Springs of Arkansas," 731.

131. James C. Minor, "The Nation's Ward; Or, Practicing Hydrotherapy at Our Greatest Health Resort," *Medical Review of Reviews* 23:5 (1917): 330, 334.

132. Minor, "The Nation's Ward," 334; M. F. Lautman, "Studies on the Physiological Action of the Natural Radioactive Water of Hot Springs, Arkansas," *Southwestern Medicine* 8:9 (1924): 437.

133. For the secondary literature on radium's therapeutic uses, see Bettyann Kevles, *Naked to the Bone: Medical Imaging in the Twentieth Century* (New Brunswick, NJ: Rutgers University Press, 1997); Claudia Clark, *Radium Girls: Women and Industrial Health Reform, 1910–1935* (Chapel Hill: University of North Carolina Press, 1997); Carolyn Thomas de la Peña, "Recharging at the Fordyce: Confronting the Machine and Nature in the Modern Bath," *Technology and Culture* 40:4 (1999): 746–69; Charles Hayter, *An Element of Hope: Radium and the Response to Cancer in Canada, 1900–1940* (Toronto: McGill-Queen's University, 2005); and Luis Campos, "The Birth of Living Radium," *Representations* 97:1 (2007): 1–27. For contemporary references to radium in the treatment of syphilis, see Frank E. Simpson, *Radium Therapy* (St. Louis, MO: C. V. Mosby, 1922): 286; Winfield Ayres, "The Effect of Intravenous Injection of Radium on a Persistent Positive Wassermann Reaction," *Radium* 6:3 (1915): 57–59; and George M. MacKee, *X-Rays and Radium in the Treatment of Diseases of the Skin* (New York: Lea and Febiger, 1921), 509.

134. Granville MacGowan, "The Treatment of Syphilis," *Therapeutic Gazette* 30:8 (1906): 518; "County Editors in Little Rock," *Fourth Estate*, June 1, 1918, 8; William Augustus Hardaway, *Handbook of Cutaneous Disease* (New York: Lea Brothers, 1907), 504; "Radioactivity of the Waters at Hot Springs, Ark., and Saratoga Springs, New York, and Other Points in America," *Radium* 5:1 (1915): 10–11; William P. Headden, "The Doughty Springs, as a Group of Radium-Bearing Springs on the South Fork of the Gunnisan River, Delta County, Colorado," *Proceedings of the Colorado Scientific Society*, vol. 8 (Denver: Colorado Scientific Society, 1908), 27.

135. Thomas J. Allen, "Does Water Cure?" *Medical Standard* 36:10 (1913): 386.

136. Scully, "The Role of Radio Activity of Natural Spring Waters as a Therapeutic Agent," 211.

137. Scully, "The Role of Radio Activity of Natural Spring Waters as a Therapeutic Agent," 211.

138. Scully, "The Role of Radio Activity of Natural Spring Waters as a Therapeutic Agent," 208.

139. Scully, "The Role of Radio Activity of Natural Spring Waters as a Therapeutic Agent," 208.

140. Scully, "The Role of Radio Activity of Natural Spring Waters as a Therapeutic Agent," 211, 208.

141. Scully, "The Role of Radio Activity of Natural Spring Waters as a Therapeutic Agent," 211.

142. Scully, "The Role of Radio Activity of Natural Spring Waters as a Therapeutic Agent," 211–12.

143. Holland, "The Use of Radioactive Waters," 1108.

144. Minor, "Water, the Main Factor in the Prevention of Disease," 345.

145. L. M. Maus, "A Sketch of the Hot Springs of Arkansas, America's National Health Resort," *Journal of the Arkansas Medical Society* 21:3 (1924): 55.

146. For examples of some of the ways in which American medical practitioners made use of Wagner-Jauregg's novel treatment, see Joel T. Braslow, *Mental Ills and Bodily Cures: Psychiatric Treatment in the First Half of the Twentieth Century* (Berkeley: University of California Press, 1997), esp. chapter 5; and Margaret Humphreys, "Whose Body? Whose Disease? Studying Malaria while Treating Neurosyphilis," in *Useful Bodies: Humans in the Service of Medical Science in the Twentieth Century* (Baltimore, MD: Johns Hopkins Press, 2003), 53–80.

147. Jay F. Schamberg and Thomas Butterworth, "Diathermy in the Treatment of General Paralysis and in Wassermann-Fast Syphilis," *American Journal of Syphilis* 16:4 (1932): 519–20. For evidence of the search for alternatives to malaria therapy, see J. C. King and E. W. Cocke, "Therapeutic Fever Produced by Diathermy with Special Reference to Its Application in the Treatment of Paresis," *Southern Medical Journal* 23:3 (1930): 222–28; C. A. Neymann and S. L. Osborne, "The Treatment of Dementia Paralytica with Hyperpyrexia Produced by Diathermy," *Journal of the American Medical Association* 96:22 (1931): 7–11; W. L. Wilson, "Clinical Use of Fever in the Treatment of Syphilis," *Military Surgeon* 72:4 (1933): 292–96; Walter M. Simpson, "Artificial Fever Therapy," *Journal of the American Medical Association* 105:26 (1935): 2132–40; and Paul O' Leary et al., "Malaria and Artificial Fever in the Treatment of Paresis," *Journal of the American Medical Association* 115:9 (1940): 677–81.

148. Schamberg and Butterworth, "Diathermy in the Treatment of General Paralysis and in Wassermann-Fast Syphilis," 532.

149. Thompson, "Some of the Unresolved Problems of Syphilis," 52–53.

150. Purdum, "The Thermal Baths in the Treatment of Syphilis," 137.

151. Purdum, "The Thermal Baths in the Treatment of Syphilis," 138.

152. For an example of this, see *Thirteenth Biennial Report of the State Board of Health of the State of Mississippi* (Jackson, MS: State Board of Health, 1935), 181.

153. "Hot Bath" in *The Practitioners Library of Medicine and Surgery*, vol. 8: *Therapeutics* (New York: Appleton, 1938), 92.

154. Purdum, "The Thermal Baths in the Treatment of Syphilis," 139.

155. G. Allison Hinton, "Echinacea, Phtyolacca, Iris, and Vegetable Alternatives in the Treatment of Syphilis," *National Eclectic Medical Association* 1 (1909): 116.

156. "Recovery from Severe Syphilis without Medicine," *Journal of Venereal Disease Information* 18:8 (1937): 306; J. F. Briscoe, "A Discussion on Syphilis with Special Reference to (A) Its Prevalence and Intensity in the Past and at the Present Day; (B) Its Relation to Public Health, Including Congenital Syphilis; (C) the Treatment of the Disease," in *Proceedings of the Royal Society of Medicine*, general reports, vol. 5 (London: Longman, Green, 1912), 108. See also "Syphilis Treated and Untreated," *Medical Critic and Guide* 29 (September 1931): 281.

157. Jean Dardel, "Mineral Water Methods in the Treatment of Syphilis," *Urologic and Cutaneous Review*, Technical Supplement 2:4 (1914): 295. See also J. H. Tilden, *Gonorrhea and Syphilis: A Drugless Treatment of Venereal Disease*, 2nd ed. (Denver, CO: Smith Brooks Press, 1912).

158. Robert E. McNamara, *Chiropractic: Other Drugless Healing Methods with Criticism of the Practice of Medicine* (Davenport, IA: Wagner's Printery, 1913), 237.

159. "Medical Fiddlers," *Health Culture* 23:11 (1917): 512.

160. Louis von Cotzhausen, "Electric and Other Drugless Treatments of Locomotor Ataxia," *Monthly Cyclopedia and Medical Bulletin* 6:8 (1913): 465.

161. Aaron Kern, "The Treatment of Syphilis without Drugs," *American Journal of Physiologic Therapeutics* 1:4 (1910): 204.

162. C. Brooks Willmott, "Treatment of Syphilis," *Kentucky Medical Journal* 25:2 (1927): 63. The speaker in question here was named Edward R. Palmer.

163. Willmott, "Treatment of Syphilis," 63.

164. Willmott, "Treatment of Syphilis," 60. The speaker in question here was a doctor named Curran Pope.

165. Willmott, "Treatment of Syphilis," 60.

166. Willmott, "Treatment of Syphilis," 61.

167. Darnel, "Mineral Water Methods," 296.

168. Charles C. Dennie and Albert N. Lemoine, "An Efficient Method of Heat Therapy in the Treatment of Syphilis," *Journal of the Missouri Medical Association* 31:5 (1934): 185.

169. Dennie and Lemoine, "An Efficient Method of Heat Therapy in the Treatment of Syphilis," 187, 189.

170. *Kansas City Medical Journal* 13 (1937): 14.

171. C.A. Owens, "Fever Therapy in the Treatment of Gonorrhea," *Nebraska State Medical Journal* 23:8 (1938): 308.

172. Wenger, "A Study of Hydrotherapy in Relation to the Treatment of Syphilis," 323.

173. Wenger, "A Study of Hydrotherapy in Relation to the Treatment of Syphilis," 324.

174. Wenger, "A Study of Hydrotherapy in Relation to the Treatment of Syphilis," 327.

175. Elmer Lee, "Medical Democracy," *North American Journal of Homeopathy* 67:5 (1919): 472.

176. Wooton, "The Adequate Treatment of Syphilis," 95.

177. Minor, "The Nation's Ward," 330, 334.

178. Minor, "Water, the Main Factor in the Prevention of Disease," 80.

Epilogue

1. "VD Commended," *Arkansas Health Bulletin* 6:8 (1949): 3.

2. "VD Control in Arkansas," *Arkansas Health Bulletin* 2:8 (1945): 4–5.

3. Thomas N. Meroney and Daniel D. Swinney, "Your V.D. Control Registry," *Arkansas Health Bulletin* 1:7 (1944): 5–7.

4. "Venereal Disease Control," *Arkansas Health Bulletin* 1:3 (1944): 6–9.

5. The second verse of this song's lyrics read as follows: "A ranch on the range isn't likely to find / Much use for a cowboy who's dead, lame, or blind / So if you've known Katey, please listen to this: / Only a doctor can cure syphilis! / Don't be / an ignorant cowboy / an ignorant, ignorant cowboy" ("All Set to Spin," *Arkansas Health Bulletin* 6:9 [1949]: 1).

6. In 1945, the state officially registered 13,403 cases of acquired syphilis. By 1950, the annual incidence of syphilis within Arkansas had fallen to 6,145 cases ("Syphilis in Arkansas, 1945–1950," *Arkansas Health Bulletin* 8:7 [1951]: 8).

7. For more on this development, see John Parascandola, "Quarantining Women: Venereal Disease Rapid Treatment Centers in World War Two America," *Bulletin of the History of Medicine* 83:3 (2009): 431–59.

8. "VD Summarizes Fiscal Year, 1945–46," *Arkansas Health Bulletin* 3:10 (1946): 2.

9. Meroney and Swinney, "Your V.D. Control Registry," 7.

10. The establishment of "rapid treatment centers" in other states played a significant role in this process. After the city of St. Louis constructed such a facility, for example, medical authorities reported that only a "limited number of neurosyphilis patients" were being transferred to Hot Springs for treatment. See Kansas State Board of Health, *Biennial Report* 23 (Topeka, KS: Ferd Voiland Jr., 1948), 65.

11. For these references, see G. E. Parkhurst, "Treatment of Neurosyphilis at Hot Springs V.D. Medical Center," in *Recent Advances in the Study of Venereal Diseases* (Washington, DC: Venereal Disease Education Institute, 1949), 209–16; H. Eisenberg, M. R. Davis, L. S. Wright, and E. B. Johnwick, "Electrocardiographic Changes in Secondary Syphilis," *American Journal of Syphilis, Gonorrhea, and Venereal Diseases* 36:5 (1952): 418–22; and T. E. Osmond, G. E. Parkhurst, F. W. Harb, and G. R. Cannefax, "Penicillin-Resistant Gonorrhea vs. Nonspecific Urethritis" *Journal of Venereal Disease Information* 28:10 (1947): 211–14.

12. For evidence of this, see *United States Public Health Service Medical Center, Hot Springs, Arkansas* (Little Rock, AR: Arkansas State Board of Health, 1952).

13. See Nelda King, "Pool Therapy," *Tri-State Medical Journal* 4:8 (1930): 905; Maurice F. Lautman, "Hydrotherapy in the Treatment of Arthritis," *Journal of the Arkansas Medical Society* 29:4 (1932): 94–96; Louis G. Martin, "Under Water Physiotherapy and Pool Therapy," *Journal of the Arkansas Medical Society* 30:11 (1934): 229–31; and Euclid M. Smith, "Underwater Therapy in the Treatment of Chronic Arthritis," *Journal of the Arkansas Medical Society* 32:9 (1936): 137–38.

14. George M. Fletcher, "The Place of Health Resort Therapy in the Treatment of Conditions Affecting the General Nervous System," *Tri-State Medical Journal* 15:6 (1943): 2919.

15. Euclid M. Smith and Charles H. Lutterloh, "Spa Therapy in Rheumatic Diseases," *Archives of Physical Therapy* 21:3 (1940): 142.

16. Smith and Lutterloh, "Spa Therapy in Rheumatic Diseases," 143.

17. Francis J. Scully, "The Role of Radio Activity of Natural Spring Waters as a Therapeutic Agent," *Journal of the Arkansas Medical Society* 30:11 (1934): 212.

18. Euclid M. Smith, "Health Resort Therapy in the United States," *Transactions of the American Therapeutic Society* 151 (1941): 79.

19. For evidence of local doctors' lack of interest in this disease, see Francis J. Scully, "Spa Therapy of Arthritis and Rheumatic Disorders," *Archives of Physical Medicine* 26:4 (1945): 233–38.

20. For more on this, see Roy Porter, *Blood and Guts: A Short History of Medicine* (New York: Norton, 2002), 107.

21. For an account of the decline of these health resorts, see Gregg Mitman, *Breathing Space: How Allergies Shape our Lives and Landscapes* (New Haven, CT: Yale University Press, 1997).

22. Edwina Walls, "The Public Health Service VD Clinic in Hot Springs, AR," *Public Health Reports* 110:1 (1995): 103–4.

23. Oliver C. Wenger, "Results of a Study and Investigation of Venereal Disease at the U.S. Public Health Service Clinic at Hot Springs, Arkansas," Oliver C. Wenger Papers, University of Arkansas for Medical Sciences Archives.

24. For a good example of this trend, see Elizabeth Fee, "Science v. Sin: Venereal Disease in Baltimore in the Twentieth Century," *Journal of the History of Medicine and Allied Sciences* 43:2 (1988): 141–64.

25. As evidence of changing public attitudes toward VD, consider a public service announcement published in the *Arkansas Health Bulletin* in 1945. Announcing the opening of a new nightclub called "Charcot's Joint," the advertisement's tone is remarkable for its comedic, destigmatized treatment of syphilis and gonorrhea. Located in "Chancre Heights," the club's address was listed as "606 Salvarsan Boulevard." The club's house band was named "Lues Gumma and His Condyloma Orchestra," and the evening's performance featured "Four Plus Wassermann and his Argile Robertson Pupils." "Always a Congenital Crowd," the billboard boasted, adding "Paresis Reasonable," "Attaxis Included," and "Tabes for Ladies." See *Arkansas Health Bulletin* 2:8 (1945): 131.

26. For a discussion of these trends in another geographical context, see Monica Dux, "'A More Enlightened Approach?' Venereal Disease Legislation in Post-World War Two Australia," *Melbourne Historical Journal* 29 (February 2001): 64–70.

27. For more on this, see Alan Ingram, "Domopolitics and Disease: HIV/AIDS, Immigration, and Asylum in the UK," *Environment and Planning D: Society and Space* 26:5 (2008): 875–94.

28. In 2015, the prominent right-wing British politician Nigel Farage fueled this ongoing controversy after erroneously claiming that the United Kingdom's National Health Service was annually spending roughly £2 billion on antiretroviral drugs for HIV-positive foreigners. See Patrick Butler, "Do Foreigners Come to the UK to Get HIV Treatment?" *Guardian*, April 3, 2015.

Page numbers in *italics* refer to figures and tables.